Cataract

ESASO Course Series

Vol. 3

Series Editors

F. Bandello Milan
B. Corcóstegui Barcelona

Cataract

Volume Editor

José L. Güell Barcelona

178 figures, 168 in color, and 5 tables, 2013

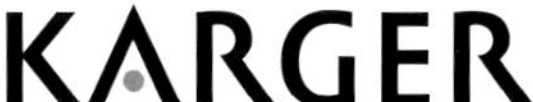

Basel · Freiburg · Paris · London · New York · New Delhi · Bangkok · Beijing · Tokyo · Kuala Lumpur · Singapore · Sydney

José L. Güell
Director of Cornea and Refractive Surgery Unit
Instituto Microcirugía Ocular (IMO)
President of EuCornea (European Society of Cornea
and Ocular Disease Specialists)
Associate Professor of Ophthalmology
Universidad Autónoma de Barcelona
C/ Josep Ma Lladó, 3
ES–08035 Barcelona (Spain)

Library of Congress Cataloging-in-Publication Data

Cataract (2013)
 Cataract / volume editor, José L. Güell.
    p. ; cm. -- (ESASO course series, ISSN 1664-882X ; vol. 3)
 At head of title: Selected contributions from ESASO modules 2009 and 2010
 Includes bibliographical references and indexes.
 ISBN 978-3-318-02410-4 (hard cover : alk. paper) -- ISBN 978-3-318-02411-1 (electronic version)
 I. Güell, José L., 1960- editor of compilation. II. European School for Advanced Studies in
Ophthalmology, issuing body. III. Title. IV. Title: Selected contributions from ESASO modules 2009
and 2010. V. Series: ESASO course series ; v. 3. 1664-882X
 [DNLM: 1. Cataract. 2. Cataract Extraction--methods. 3. Lenses, Intraocular. 4. Refractive Surgical
Procedures--methods. WW 260]
 RE451
 617.7'42059--dc23

                                                                              2013021128

Bibliographic Indices. This publication is listed in bibliographic services, including Current Contents®.

© Copyright 2013 by S. Karger AG, P.O. Box, CH–4009 Basel (Switzerland)
www.karger.com
Printed in Germany on acid-free and non-aging paper (ISO 9706) by Kraft Druck, Ettlingen
ISSN 1664–882X
e-ISSN 1664–8838
ISBN 978–3–318–02410–4
eISBN 978–3–318–02411–1

Contents

List of Contributors

Roberto Bellucci
Chief of Hospital Ophthalmology
Hospital and University of Verona
Borgo Trento Hospital
IT–37126 Verona (Italy)
E-Mail roberto.bellucci@ospedaleuniverona.it

Lucio Buratto
Centro Ambrosiano Oftalmico
Piazza della Repubblica 21
IT–20124 Milan (Italy)
E-Mail iol.lasik@buratto.com

Myriam Cassagne
Department of Ophthalmology
Purpan Hospital
Place du Dr Baylac
FR–31059 Toulouse (France)
E-Mail iol.lasik@buratto.com

Daniel Elies
Instituto Microcirugía Ocular
Universidad Autónoma de Barcelona
Josep Maria Lladó, 3
ES–08035 Barcelona (Spain)
E-Mail elies@imo.es

Oscar Gris
Instituto Microcirugía Ocular
Universidad Autónoma de Barcelona
Josep Maria Lladó, 3
ES–08035 Barcelona (Spain)
E-Mail gris@imo.es

Jose. L. Güell
Instituto Microcirugía Ocular
Universidad Autónoma de Barcelona
Josep Maria Lladó, 3
ES–08035 Barcelona (Spain)
E-Mail guell@imo.es

François Malecaze
Department of Ophthalmology
Purpan Hospital
FR–31024 Toulouse (France)
E-Mail malecaze.fr@chu-toulouse.fr

Felicidad Manero
Instituto Microcirugía Ocular
Universidad Autónoma de Barcelona
Josep Maria Lladó, 3
ES–08035 Barcelona (Spain)
E-Mail manero@imo.es

Merce Morral
Instituto Microcirugía Ocular
Universidad Autónoma de Barcelona
Josep Maria Lladó, 3
ES–08035 Barcelona (Spain)
E-Mail merce.morral@gmail.com

Zoltan Z. Nagy
Department of Ophthalmology
Semmelweis University
Maria u. 39
HU–1085 Budapest (Hungary)
E-Mail zoltan.nagy100@gmail.com

Ioannis G. Pallikaris
Department of Ophthalmology
Medical School
University of Crete
71003 Heraklion, Crete (Greece)
E-Mail pallikar@med.uoc.gr

Marie Porterie
Department of Ophthalmology
Purpan Hospital
Place du Dr Baylac
FR–31059 Toulouse (France)
E-Mail pallikar@med.uoc.gr

Khiun Tjia
Isala Clinics
Groot Wezenland 20
8011JW Zwolle (The Netherlands)
E-Mail kftjia@gmail.com

Paula Verdaguer
Instituto Microcirugía Ocular
Universidad Autónoma de Barcelona
Josep Maria Lladó, 3
ES–08035 Barcelona (Spain)
E-Mail paulaverdaguer@gmail.com

Preface

Today, there are multiple attractive options for postgraduate training in ophthalmology, but at the same time, it is frequently confusing for the surgeon to select the best one, taking into account the time and space limitations we all need to deal with. Focused peer-reviewed journals, specialized books, national and international meetings and courses, multiple specialized and more general websites, etc., are all useful but they have their own and particular limitations: sometimes they are already a little bit outdated when they reach us, sometimes they are disorganized, and sometimes it is inconvenient to attend proper meetings or meetings that receive low scientific and academic support. This is why some European societies are strongly focusing on investing their time and instruments in education, as is the case with the ESCRS and EuCornea.

Following our experience and excellent response from the participants through the teaching modules in Lugano, the main goal of the ESASO Course Series has been to offer to the ophthalmology trainee an update review of a selection of important topics, mixing basic information with the most advanced techniques. In this book, the authors of each lesson are world-renowned surgeons who spend a significant amount of their time teaching and sharing their own experience with academicism and generosity. We all hope you enjoy this first volume on cataract and refractive surgery.

Jose L. Güell, Barcelona

Güell JL (ed): Cataract. ESASO Course Series. Basel, Karger, 2013, vol 3, pp 1–25
DOI: 10.1159/000350899

Cataract Surgery: An Update on Basics and Surgical Tips

Khiun Tjia

Isala Clinics, Zwolle, The Netherlands

Abstract

In this chapter, the basics of fluidics and ultrasound action are rehearsed, which are fundamental to better understand the challenges and solutions of all kinds of non-routine phacoemulsification cases. Specific properties of torsional ultrasound are explained, which give a better insight of the advantages of this ultrasound modality. Practical tips and tricks are provided to improve one's hydrodissection skills, soft lens removal and the pitfalls of posterior polar cataract. Hard cataracts and chop techniques are thoroughly discussed as well as small pupil management. Challenging situations such as mature and hypermature cataracts, floppy iris syndrome, weak zonules and last but not least posterior capsule rupture management are explained.

This chapter is intended to refresh the study material provided at the ESASO cataract module by the author, Khiun Tjia, a cataract surgery specialist. This reading material is not suitable as a stand-alone educational tool, but should be combined with the video clips presented during the course.

The information in this chapter reflects my opinion of cataract surgery techniques. It only covers the topics discussed during the one-day course by Dr. Tjia.

There are many textbooks on cataract surgery, which can help the reader understand cataract surgery technology and techniques in depth.

Basics Fluidics and Ultrasound

The key point in fluid dynamics during phacoemulsification surgery is that the fluid going into the eye should always exceed the amount of fluid going out of the eye at all times. If not, the anterior chamber shallows and the posterior capsule will move upward and potentially come into contact with the phacotip, which can result in a posterior capsule rupture.

The inflow is determined by the irrigation flow only; the hydrostatic pressure of the water column in the irrigation line until the level of the drip chamber underneath the infusion bottle is expressed in centimeters (bottle height). The resistance in the entire irrigation line including the narrow space between the sleeve and the phacotip determines the final irrigation flow: irrigation pressure/irrigation resistance.

When the phacotip is completely occluded, and no leak flow occurs through any of the incisions, one must be aware of the actual intraocular pressure. The entire fluid (water) column of the irrigation line presses in the eye. For instance, a

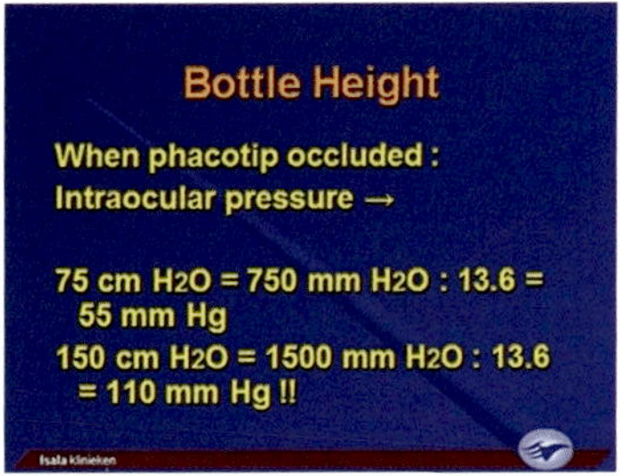

Fig. 1. Bottle height.

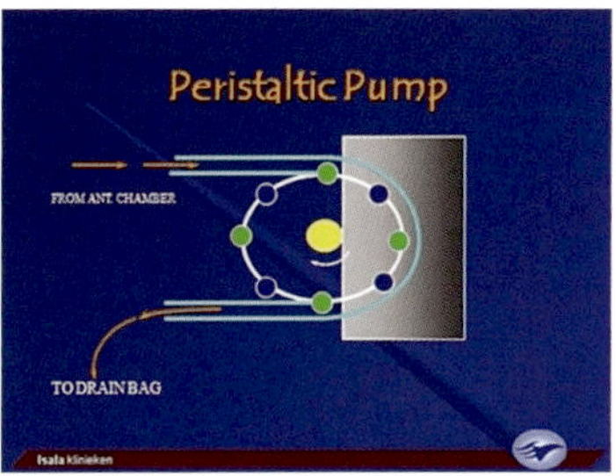

Fig. 2. Peristaltic pump.

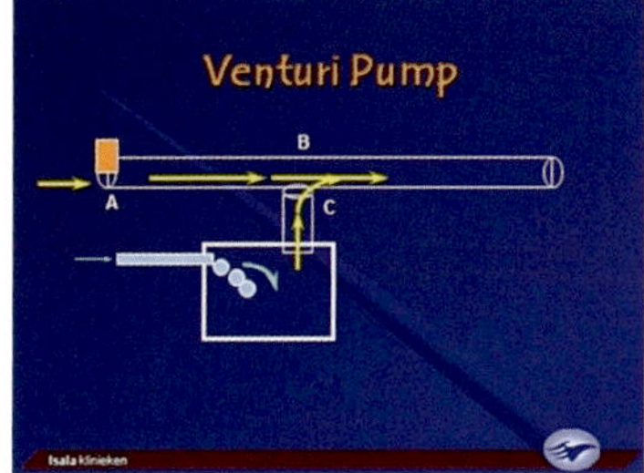

Fig. 3. Venturi pump.

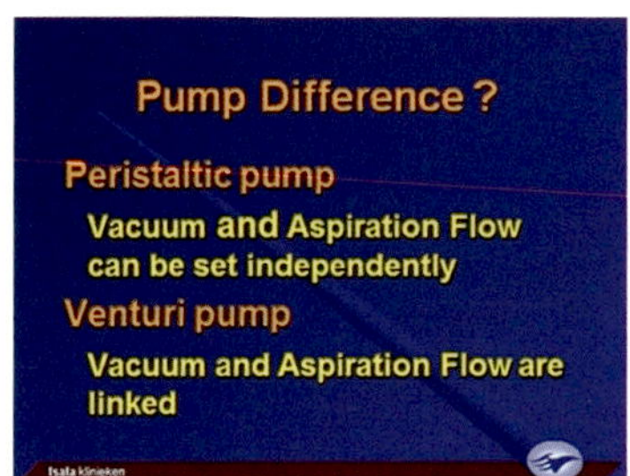

Fig. 4. Pump difference.

bottle height of 75 cm H_2O translates into 750 mm H_2O, and divided by the relative weight of mercury of 13.6 results in an intraocular pressure of approximately 55 mm Hg. Extreme bottle heights of 150 cm are used by some surgeons, which results in 110 mm Hg pressure when the tip is occluded (fig. 1)! One should be extremely cautious about utilizing bottle heights exceeding 100 cm which causes pressure spikes of more than 73 mm Hg.

Irrigation pressure is either passive with a bottle hanging above the level of the eye as described above, or is active by a pressurized system, which is not discussed in this chapter. With an active pressure system, the required pressure can be set on the machine in mm Hg.

Before discussing outflow, we have to understand the different pump systems of existing phacomachines: peristaltic pump systems and Venturi pump systems.

Peristaltic pumps consist of rollers which push fluid through a flexible aspiration tubing. The aspiration flow increases with the increasing speed of the rollers (fig. 2).

Venturi pumps create a vacuum in a rigid cassette by forcing gas through a pipe connected to the cassette. With more gas force blown through the pipe, higher vacuum is created in the cassette, which in turn attracts more fluid from the aspiration line (fig. 3).

The main difference between the two systems is that in Venturi pump systems, the vacuum and aspiration flow are directly linked to each other. One cannot set a high vacuum and a low flow. With a peristaltic pump, vacuum and aspiration flow can be controlled independently (fig. 4).

Outflow of the eye during phacosurgery is more complex and consists of the following: aspiration flow, leak flow and surge flow.

As a cataract surgery specialist, I have a very specific preference for peristaltic pump systems. The ability to control vacuum and flow separately is essential for managing challenging cases for me. I am discussing fluidic dynamics in the peristaltic machine in the next paragraph.

Aspiration Flow
The speed of rollers in the cassette determines the aspiration flow and can be set on the machine in ml/min. Aspiration flow can only occur when the tip is not fully obstructed. When the phacotip is fully occluded, there is no flow. The actual flow passing through the aspiration line is dependent on the force of the phacopump pulling the fluid, and the total resistance in the aspiration line. Pump capacities and aspiration line lumen sizes vary among the available phacomachines. The preset values displayed on the machines do not necessarily occur in real time. A good example is that the aspiration flow at the same machine setting of e.g. 50 ml/min can be close to that value with a large bore phacotip of 0.7 mm and a normally large lumen aspiration tubing. In contrast, the preset value of 50 ml/min will not be reached through the very small 0.3-mm port of the I/A aspiration port opening. This can be easily less than half of that value, depending on the system specifications.

Vacuum
The vacuum which is displayed on the machine is the preset maximum level. When the tip is occluded, the pump rollers will continue to spin until the preset maximum vacuum level is reached. The time necessary to reach this maximum vacuum level (vacuum rise time) is dependent on the speed of the rollers (aspiration flow setting). The same high vacuum level can be reached either at a high speed/high flow setting or at a slower pace/low flow setting. The maximum vacuum level is lost when the tip occlusion breaks. This normally happens anytime when ultrasound is activated in footswitch position 3. Vacuum is only built up in

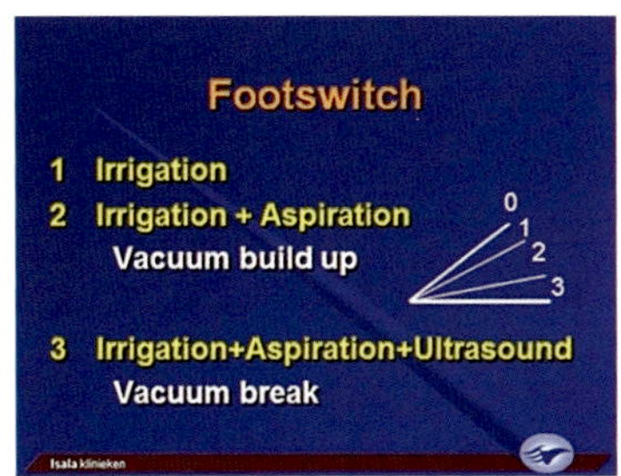

Fig. 5. Footswitch.

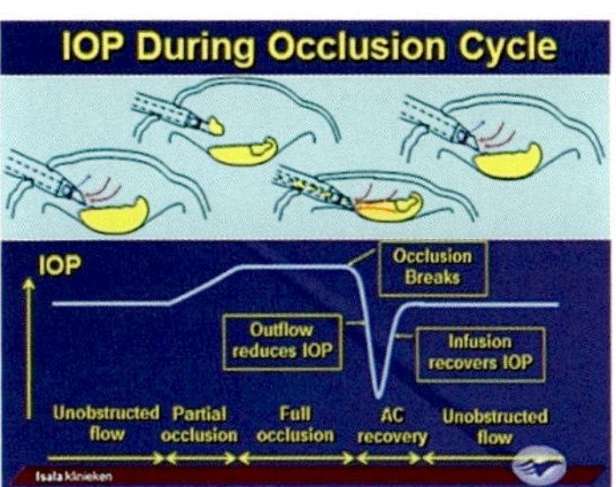

Fig. 6. Occlusion cycle.

footswitch position 2 when both irrigation and aspiration occur. (fig. 5).

Vacuum is the holding force of the machine, which keeps lens material at the tip to be emulsified and to pull the lens material through the aspiration line. There is always a debate about the required level of vacuum in phacosurgery. In essence, it can simplified by the following: high enough to do the job, but not too high because of one potential drawback. This 'drawback' phenomenon is 'surge flow'.

Surge
The mechanism of surge flow only occurs at the moment of occlusion break and vacuum loss. It is a very brief moment in a fraction of a second, when the contracted aspiration line under vacuum suddenly springs back to its original shape and volume when vacuum is lost (fig. 6–9).

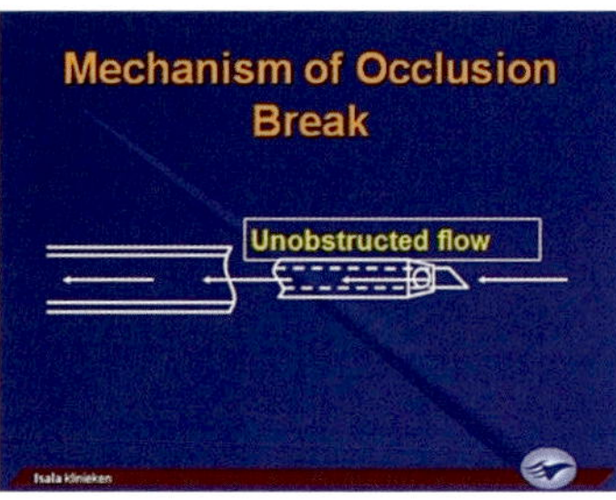

Fig. 7. Unobstructed flow.

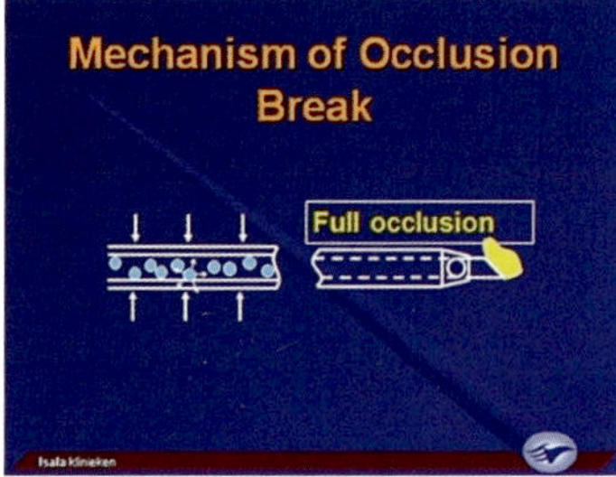

Fig. 8. Full occlusion.

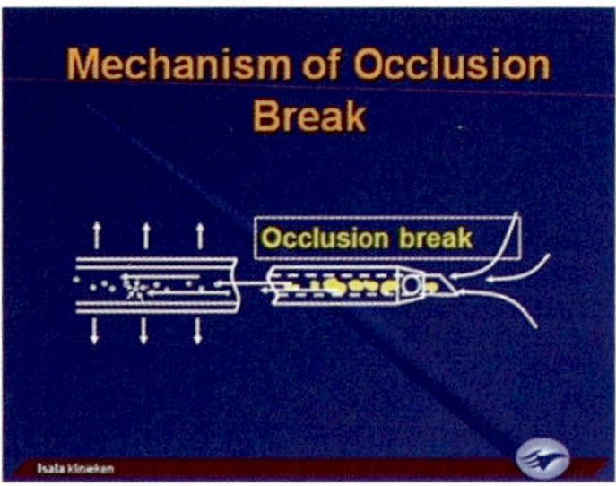

Fig. 9. Occlusion break.

The severity of the surge flow is determined by the following factors:

- Vacuum; surge increases with higher vacuum
- Phacotip lumen; a smaller lumen will restrict the amount of fluid during the surge
- Sleeve size; a larger sleeve will allow more fluid into the eye during surge
- Infusion pressure; a higher bottle will push more fluid in the eye during surge
- Compliance of tubing; softer tubing material will contract more resulting in higher surge

Beware of Air!

When a significant amount of air is inadvertently aspirated, the post-occlusion surge response can be dramatically higher because air is much more compliant than fluid. The air in the aspiration line will enlarge significantly under vacuum. On occlusion break, the air will return to its original volume, markedly adding to the force of the surge. Air is easily aspirated when the phacotip is retracted from the eye while in footswitch position 2. This happens often, and many surgeons are unaware of the danger.

If air is aspirated inadvertently, one must place the phacotip in a fluid container and aspirate fluid until the air has emptied completely from the aspiration line.

Ultrasound

In phacoemulsification surgery, ultrasound denominates the longitudinal or sideways displacement of a hollow metal phacotip at a frequency of approximately 28,000–40,000 Hz and an amplitude of approximately 0–140 μm. The direct impact of the metal tip has an emulsification effect on the lens. There is a debate whether cavitation plays an important role in phacosurgery. This is not discussed in this chapter.

Ultrasound energy dissipated in the eye can be derived from the phacotip stroke × frequency. On the various machines, ultrasound stroke is displayed in percentages with a maximum of 100%. One should know that ultrasound power settings cannot be compared between different manufacturers. In the table below, the tip stroke of earlier generation machines is shown. 20% power in one machine results in a twice or three times longer stroke than in another machine (fig. 10).

Ultrasound and Heat Production

The friction between a moving phacotip and the silicon phacosleeve induces a temperature increase, similar to rubbing hands when they are cold. The heat production is dependent on the following factors:

– Higher ultrasound power induces more heat
– Higher frequency induces more heat
– Higher duty cycle induces more heat (duty cycle is percentage 'on time'/total time)
– Higher friction between tip and sleeve induces more heat (more pressure of tip against sleeve)

Ultrasound Modulation

Ultrasound modulation has been introduced for 2 reasons: reduction of heat and reduction of repulsion.

Repulsion is the unwanted effect caused by the forward stroke of longitudinal ultrasound, which not only emulsifies the crystalline lens, but also pushes the lens away from the tip.

A simple measure to limit the repulsive effect is to set a maximum power level during the quadrant removal step. This maximum power should be set at a level when the desired emulsification is taking place without significant repulsion (fig. 11, 12).

Ultrasound modulation can be managed in two different ways, both sharing pauses between pulses of ultrasound activation, during which the nuclear fragment can come back to the tip: pulse mode and burst mode.

In the pulse mode, the duty cycle (fig. 15) is preset on the machine, and the surgeon controls phacopower with the footswitch (fig. 13). In the burst mode, the ultrasound power is preset on the machine, and the surgeon controls the pause time between ultrasound bursts with the footswitch (fig. 14).

It is a matter of preference of the surgeon whether to use either mode. There are more sophisticated hybrid modes of ultrasound modulation available on modern phacomachines, which are beyond the scope of this chapter.

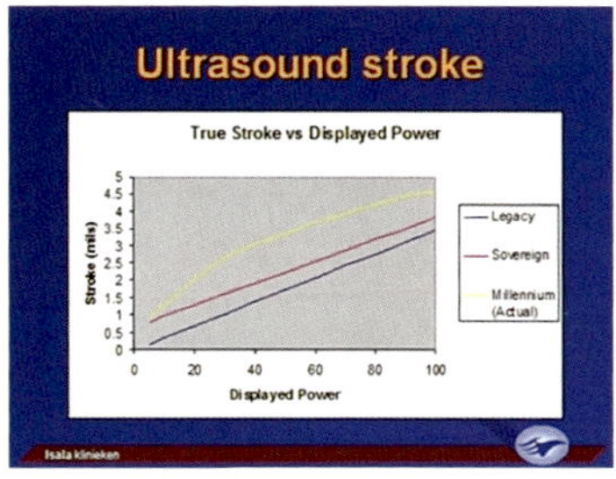

Fig. 10. Ultrasound stroke comparison.

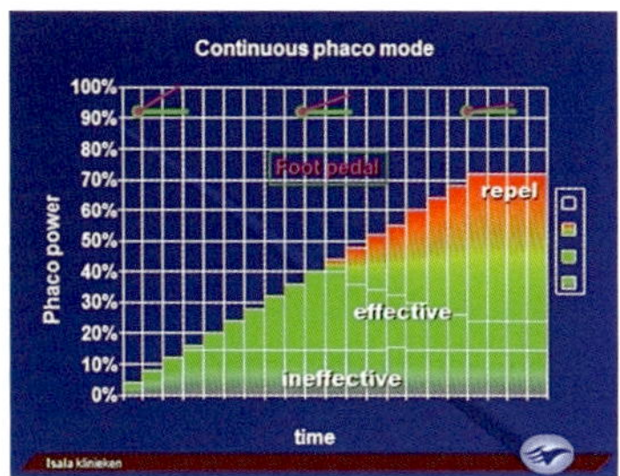

Fig. 11. Continuous mode.

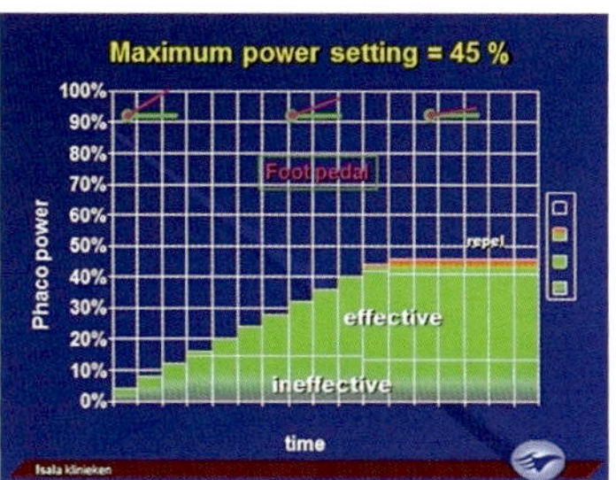

Fig. 12. Set maximum power.

Torsional Ultrasound

Torsional ultrasound technology was introduced in 2006. The mode of action is very different from traditional longitudinal ultrasound. The slight oscillatory movement of the phacotip of a Kelman style bent tip induces a sideways movement of the tip end (fig. 16). The phacotip now acts as an ultra-

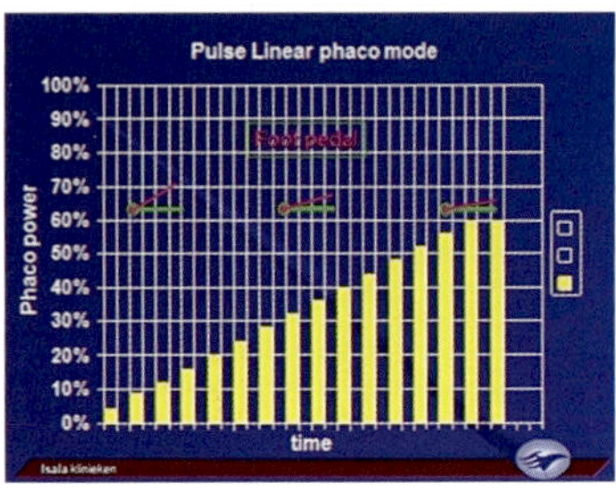

Fig. 13. Linear pulse mode.

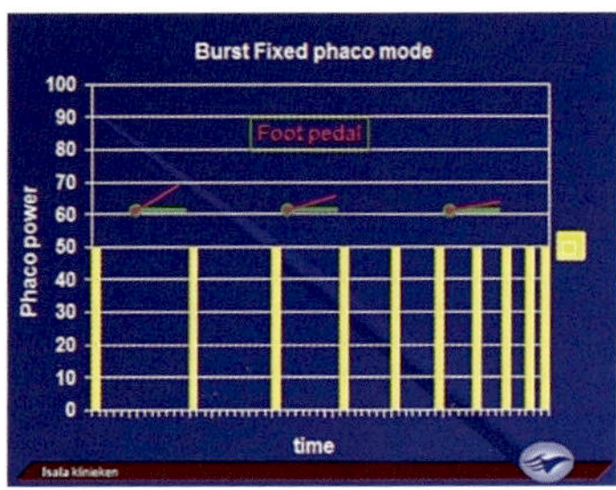

Fig. 14. Fixed burst mode.

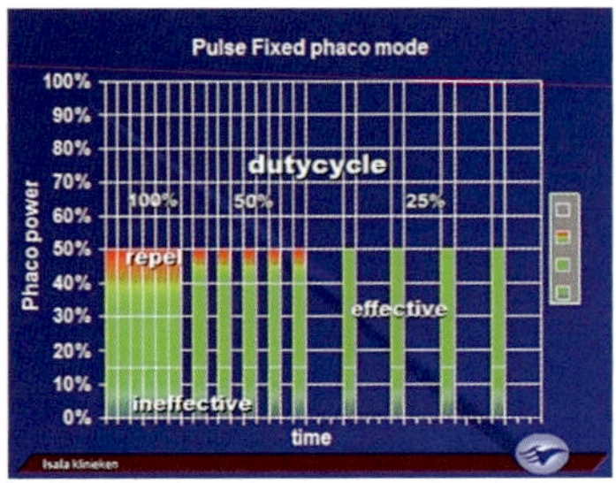

Fig. 15. Dutycycle.

sonic chafing machine instead of the ultrasonic jackhammer of longitudinal ultrasound. The main difference is that the side to side movement of the tip does not have any repulsive effect, and therefore it is more effective than traditional ultrasound. Torsional ultrasound does not require ultrasound modulation because of the lack of repulsion.

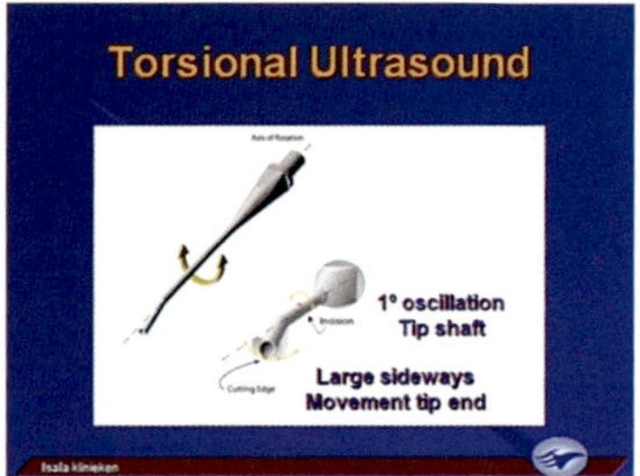

Fig. 16. Torsional ultrasound.

Transversal Ultrasound
Transversal ultrasound is combined and simultaneous action of the phacotip. The movement is elliptical, partly sideways and longitudinal. This technology can work with straight design phacotips, but tends to be also more efficient with bent tips.

OZil Tips and Tricks

Torsional ultrasound has a completely different mode of action than longitudinal ultrasound, and one should understand a few tips and tricks to experience the advantages of this technology.

In contrast to longitudinal ultrasound, which continuously repels and repositions nuclear fragments, torsional ultrasound keeps the nuclear piece right at the tip and chafes of the surface of the fragment. New lens surface has to be presented to the tip end surface for continued emulsification. For this reason, the nuclear piece has to be free to turn and tumble to emulsify efficiently. If a piece of nucleus is somehow blocked in its movement by a capsulorhexis edge, neighboring quadrant, pupil edge or sticky viscoelastic, no new lens surface can get close to the tip and emulsification stops.

Another characteristic of torsional ultrasound is that it does not give the tactile feedback of vibration as longitudinal ultrasound. And below 50% amplitude, it is hardly audible (fig. 17). Sur-

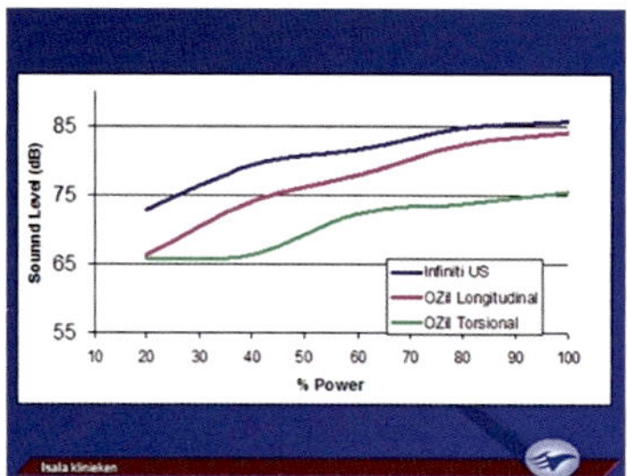

Fig. 17. Sound volume.

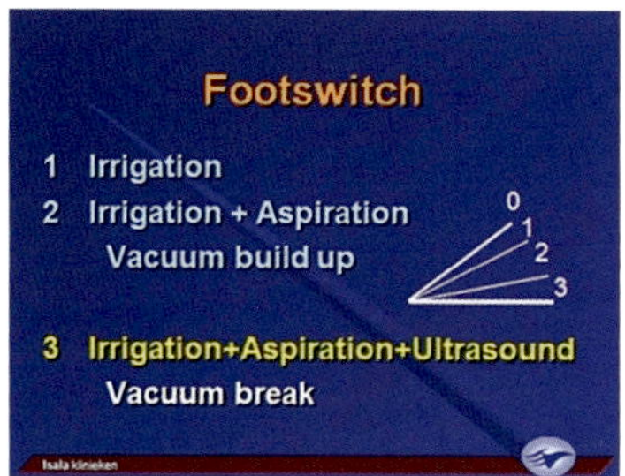

Fig. 18. Footswitch action.

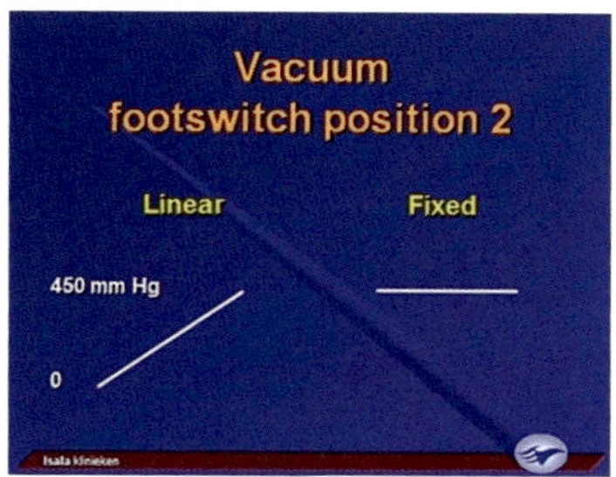

Fig. 19. Position 2.

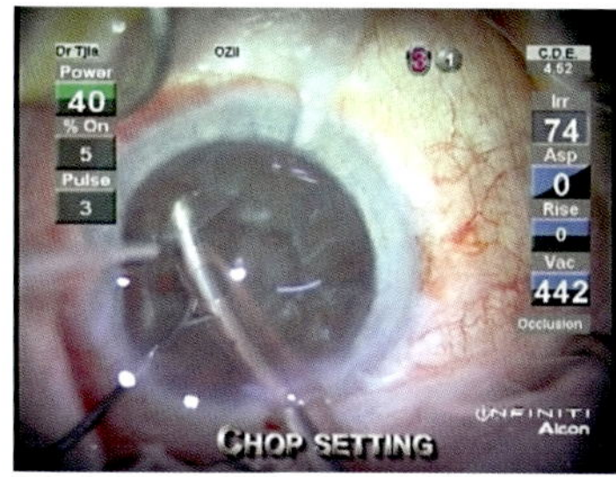

Fig. 20. Chop setting.

geons can inadvertently step into foot position 3 without hearing or feeling the activated ultrasonic action, which immediately breaks occlusion (fig. 18). To overcome this problem, one can set a louder artificial 'OZil' sound on the Infiniti machine to become aware of the foot position 3 entry.

Chop Setting
For achieving a good grip of a nuclear piece for chopping or to get a firm hold of the first quadrant after cracking the nucleus, a special 'chop' setting can be helpful. This is an extra procedure step between 'sculpt' and 'quadrant removal'. I personally recommend using longitudinal ultrasound in the pulse mode, which gives an instant tactile feedback when reaching foot position 3. I also recommend setting a high fixed vacuum, which allows the surgeon to keep a firm grip of

the quadrant in the entire range of foot position 2 (fig. 19). My personal 'chop' setting (for the Infiniti machine only; fig. 20) is: pulse mode – longitudinal US only 40% fixed, 10% duty cycle, 3 pulses/s; vacuum 450 mm Hg fixed – aspiration flow 20 ml/min.

This procedure step is only to acquire a firm grip for chopping and/or pulling a quadrant to the middle of the eye. It is not suitable for emulsification of the quadrant! This should be performed with the next procedure step 'quadrant removal'.

Torsional Ultrasound and Viscoelastic Clearing
Viscoelastic should be aspirated first to clear the space on top of the lens, prior to sculpting. Any viscoelastic can obstruct the phacotip when it drills in the lens, but dispersive viscoelastics are more sticky and should be cleared from the tip before starting to sculpt the lens. Most machines

have a default pre-phacoprocedure step with a low ultrasound setting and moderate fluidics setting only to clear the viscoelastic. If the tip is not cleared, the tip can heat too much and unwanted wound damage can occur.

Hydrodissection

There is a consensus among ophthalmologists regarding the necessity of adequate hydrodissection prior to nucleus disassembly and emulsification. For phacochop and divide-and-conquer techniques, the lens must be completely mobilized to allow easy nucleus rotation. Hydrodissection should result in a fluid wave travelling completely across the posterior surface of the lens. This ensures that complete dissection of the lens from the posterior capsule has occurred. Hydrodissection cannulas of various designs are used to accomplish the dissection.

I have noticed that many colleagues do not intentionally separate the lens from the anterior capsule. If these connections are not adequately separated, the lens will be unable to rotate. In this chapter, I describe my method for dissecting anterior capsular connections. Residents in our clinic learn this method without significant difficulty. This is a simple and logical technique that many surgeons may already practice.

Technique
After a complete posterior fluid wave crosses the entire posterior surface of the lens (fig. 21), depress the nucleus, which will subsequently separate itself from the anterior capsule at approximately the 4- or 5-o'clock position (fig. 22, 24). As you press on the nucleus, fluid underneath the nucleus will shift to the opposite side. Next, depress the nucleus on the opposite side (fig. 23, 25). The nucleus can move a little posteriorly into the accumulated fluid pool, separating itself further from the anterior capsule. If the anterior capsule remains in position when the nucleus is pressed downward close to the anterior capsulorhexis edge (fig. 4), this means that the anterior capsule and lens have separated. If one observes this separation at opposite sides of the lens, the anterior connections should be sufficiently dissected to allow easy rotation.

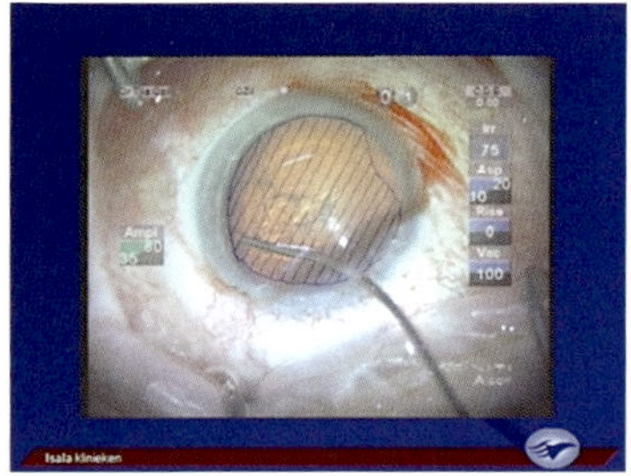

Fig. 21. Blue area = posterior wave.

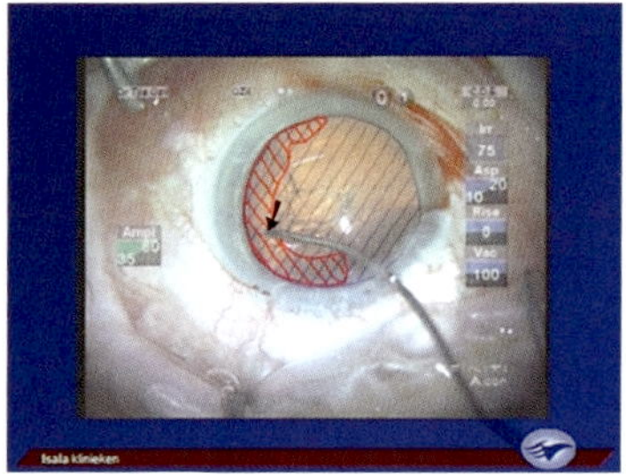

Fig. 22. Red area = anteriorly.

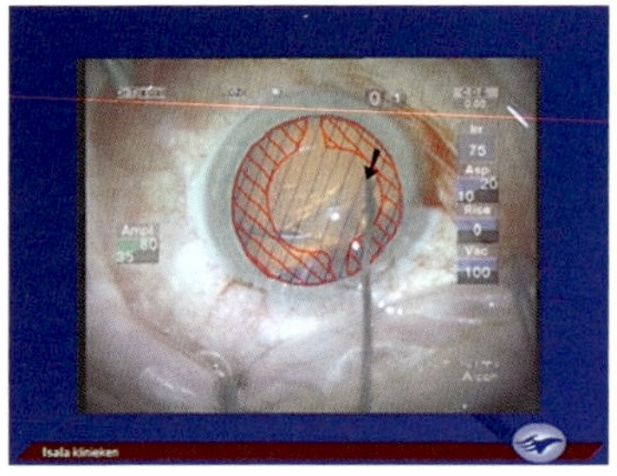

Fig. 23. 180° apart press down.

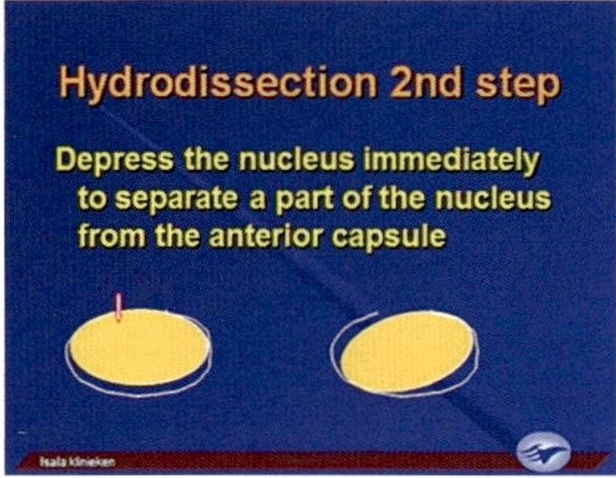

Fig. 24. Press down.

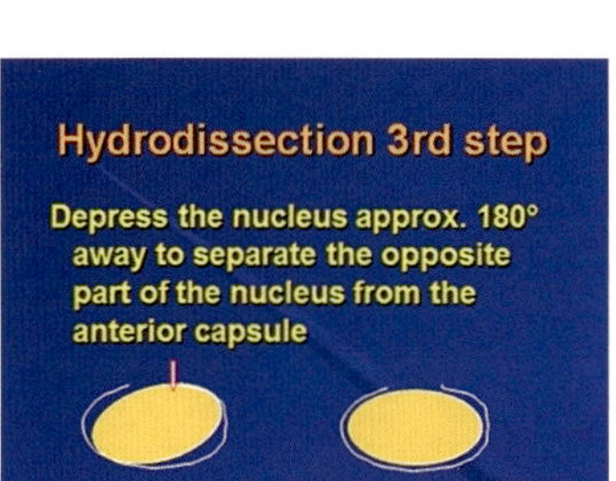

Fig. 25. Press opposite side.

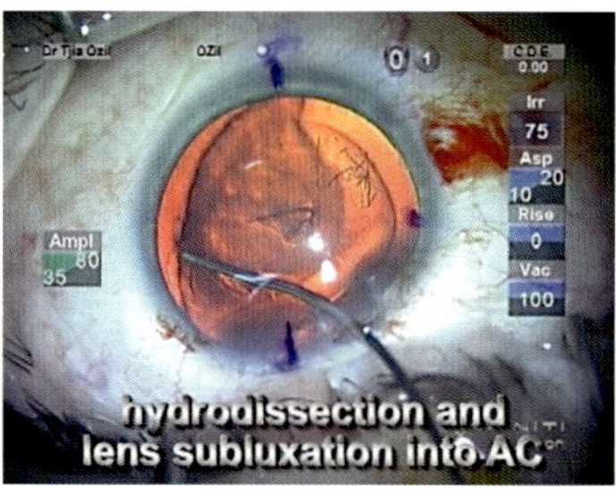

Fig. 26. Subluxate lens.

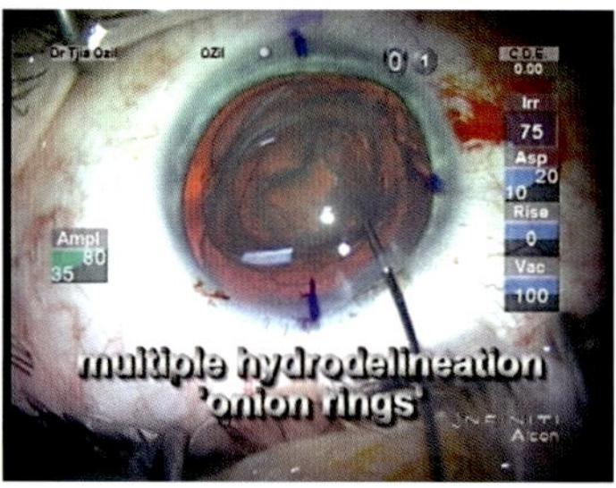

Fig. 27. Multiple hydrodelineation.

Soft Lenses

Although dense cataracts and narrow pupil cases are considered to be difficult for novice surgeons, soft lenses can be problematic for inexperienced surgeons as well. If one tries to crack or chop a soft nucleus in a conventional way, the cracking instrument does not meet any resistance and slices through the soft lens without splitting it. This can lead to repeated and unnecessary manipulations in the eye with loss of visibility and potential complications as a result.

My recommended technique for soft lens management is:
- Perform a normal hydrodissection and obtain a good cleavage plain circumferentially
- Partial subluxation of soft lens material into the anterior chamber is part of the strategy, and one should not attempt to stop or redress it (fig. 26)
- Subsequently, inject fluid in multiple cortex layers to create multi-hydrodclincation circles resembling the anatomy of an onion (fig. 27)
- Significant soft lens mass will have protruded into the anterior chamber, which facilitates the next lens removal step
- Introduce the phacotip in a bevel down position to create a direct aspiration contact with the lens
Utilize so called 'epinucleus' settings, which encompass (fig. 28):
- moderate vacuum to reduce potential surge
- moderate aspiration flow

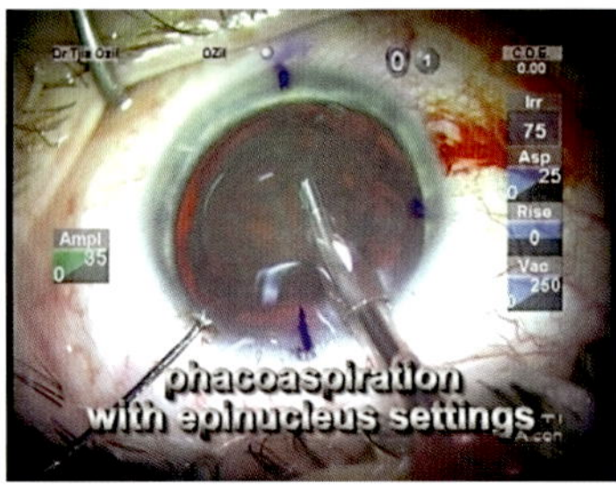

Fig. 28. Phacoaspiration.

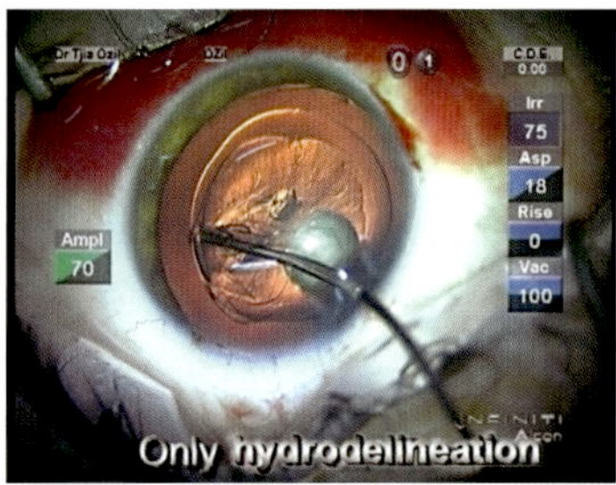

Fig. 29. No hydrodissection.

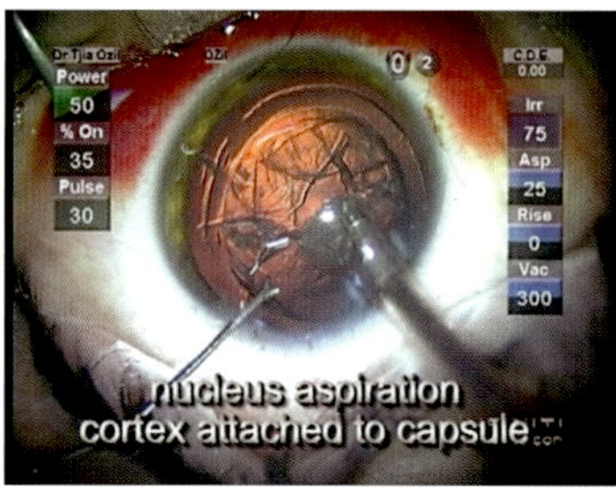

Fig. 30. Nucleus aspiration.

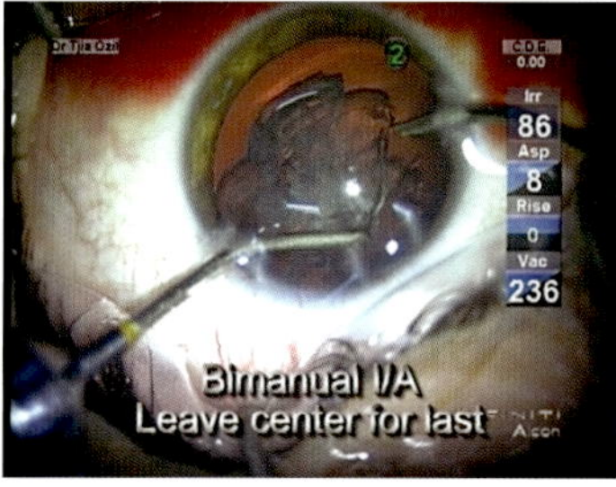

Fig. 31. Center for last.

– linear flow and vacuum settings, which enables you to very slowly aspirate the soft lens into the phacotip and as the lens is nicely molded in the tip, the footswitch can be depressed progressively to aspirate the lens
– low ultrasound power limit

The linear flow and vacuum control are essential for controlling the aspiration of a soft lens.

Posterior Polar Cataract

Posterior polar cataract cases normally only present in young patients. The soft lens management has similarities to the regular soft lens case described above.

However, there is one great caveat! The posterior pole of the lens is an extremely weak spot of the posterior capsule, which ruptures very easily. The entire strategy for handling a posterior polar cataract is based upon avoiding all potential stress to the central posterior capsule.

– No hydrodissection!
– Only hydrodelineation (fig. 29)
– A first groove can be sculpted carefully
– The soft lens halves can be aspirated, leaving the entire cortex attached to the capsule (fig. 30)
– Bimanual irrigation aspiration is preferred for easy access of the entire circumference
– Careful aspiration of peripheral cortex circumferentially, leaving the central cortex of the posterior polar zone to be aspirated at the very end (fig. 31)
– Selection of an IOL that will not cause too much stress to the posterior capsule

Hard Cataracts and Chop Techniques

For routine cataracts with soft or medium dense nuclei, I believe that all modern phacomachines are more or less equally suitable for effective and safe lens removal.

However, dense nuclei mandate significantly more ultrasonic energy prior to lens aspiration. Traditional longitudinal ultrasound intrinsically causes more repulsion with higher ultrasound power, necessitating higher vacuum and aspiration flow settings to keep the denser lens material close to the phacotip. Various strategies of ultrasound modulation have been developed to reduce the unwanted repulsive effect of longitudinal ultrasonic action.

Dispersive Viscoelastic Protection
However, the side-to-side shearing action of torsional ultrasound has proven to be more efficient and very effective at emulsifying lens material at moderate vacuum settings and very low flow aspiration flow settings.

In the longitudinal era, high vacuum settings were widely used to keep nuclear material close to the phacotip in order to increase ultrasound efficiency and decreased the required ultrasonic energy.

Even today, when using torsional ultrasound, higher vacuum settings can draw softer lens material through the phacotip and aspiration tubing without using significant ultrasonic energy levels. Dense lens material, however, needs to be completely emulsified prior to aspiration. Vacuum alone will not lead to any dense lens removal.

The key to the superior efficiency of torsional ultrasound is the absence of any intrinsic repulsive effect of the side to side shaving motion of the phacotip. Moderate vacuum is still largely sufficient to keep nuclear material at the phacotip. After emulsification of whatever density of nuclear material, the milky substance of the emulsified lens matter poses very little resistance to aspiration and therefore eliminates the need for high vacuum settings.

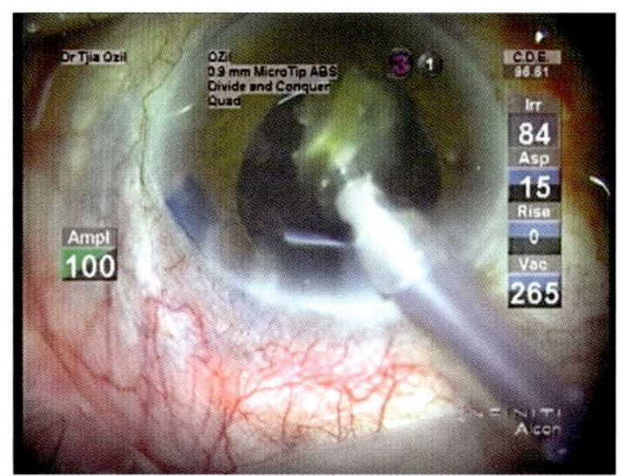

Fig. 32. Very low flow.

A very low aspiration flow (e.g. 15 ml/min) will not aspirate a dispersive viscoelastic substance that protects the corneal endothelium (fig. 32).

The combination of a dispersive viscoelastic and very low flow torsional phacoemulsification is my preferred strategy for very dense cataract surgery.

Dispersive viscoelastic substances (e.g. Viscoat®, Alcon Laboratories) are widely used to protect the corneal endothelium from the destructive effects of ultrasonic energy, fluid turbulence and/or direct impact of nuclear fragments.

The key of a low fluidics torsional phacostrategy is to leave the dispersive viscoelastic layer intact. A low aspiration flow setting is therefore mandatory to protect the fragile corneal endothelial cells.

Tip Choice for Torsional Ultrasound and Dense Nuclei
For very dense nuclei, 45° bevel tips are more efficient compared to 30° bevel tips. The 45° tips have a larger surface and make the nuclear pieces tumble around their axis whilst being emulsified. 30° tips drill more easily into the nucleus (lollipop), and emulsification halts when the sleeve obstructs further movement.

Our experience with traditional longitudinal ultrasound and very dense nuclei is that flared tip designs were prone to potential clogging of the tip. Clogging of a tip could lead to insuffi-

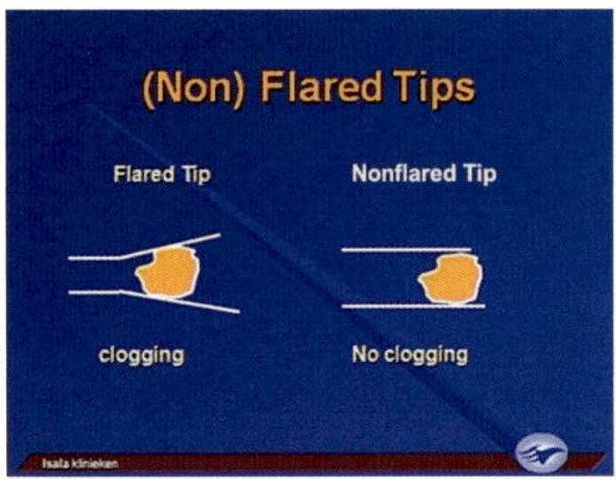

Fig. 33. Tip design.

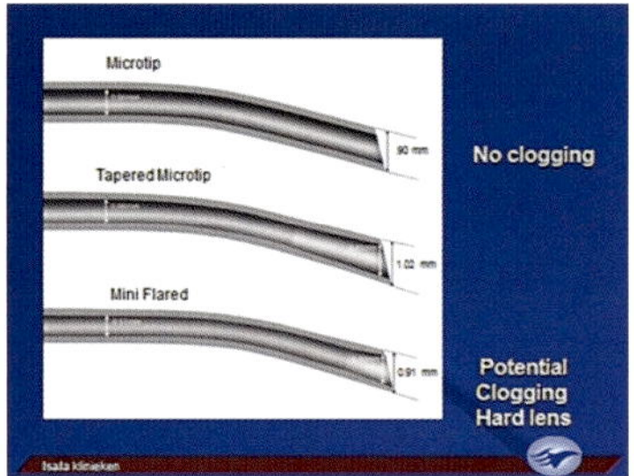

Fig. 34. Tip comparison.

cient cooling of the tip and possible heating/burn of the corneal tunnel.

Because of the sideways ultrasonic movement of a tip with torsional ultrasound, the nucleus is emulsified in a different manner. The nuclear material at the tip and inside of a flared phacotip is probably less emulsified compared to longitudinal ultrasound. There is also no significant repulsion and subsequent repositioning of the nucleus relative to the tip. This could be an explanation for the higher incidence of clogging of flared tip designs with torsional ultrasound.

Flared Tip Design and Prolonged Occlusion
The oscillatory movement of the torsional tip is highly effective in shaving lens material. However, when a flared tip design is used, the mechanism does not cause aspirated material to be 'jackhammered' into and through the tip as it is with traditional phacoemulsification. Therefore, it is important for the material to be broken up into relatively small pieces that can pass through the inner lumen of the tip without obstructing it. If torsional vibration is interrupted or larger fragments of dense lens material enter the lumen, tip obstruction may result (fig. 33, 34). These periods of prolonged tip occlusion halt the shaving process and decrease the tip efficiency.

The advantage of a bigger port opening is an increased holding surface and therefore holding power of the phacotip. With flared tips, the larger port opening narrows into a smaller size lumen shaft, which reduces the occlusion break surge. This type of flared phacotips were particularly advantageous when using longitudinal ultrasound technology, when high vacuum and aspiration flow settings were necessary to overcome the repelling effect of the longitudinal movement of the phacotip. With torsional ultrasound, lower fluidics settings are more effective and safer.

A New Nonflared Tip Design for Micro-Coaxial Phacoemulsification: The 0.9 MiniTip
Especially for denser nuclei, flared tips repeatedly show brief periods of prolonged occlusion. This can sometimes even necessitate retraction of the phacohandpiece to liberate the phacotip from nuclear material.

A new small nonflared tip has recently been introduced with an identical shaft lumen size as the MiniFlared tip of 570 μm. The outside diameter is even slightly smaller than MiniFlared tip, 800 versus 830 μm (fig. 36).

The slightly thinner wall is probably responsible for the lightly increased cutting edge tip displacement. During clinical evaluation, the 0.9 MiniTip performed very well, not showing any significant prolonged occlusion, enhancing the overall cutting efficiency, specifically for denser nuclei (fig. 37).

A comparison of the performance of several tip designs is shown in figure 35.

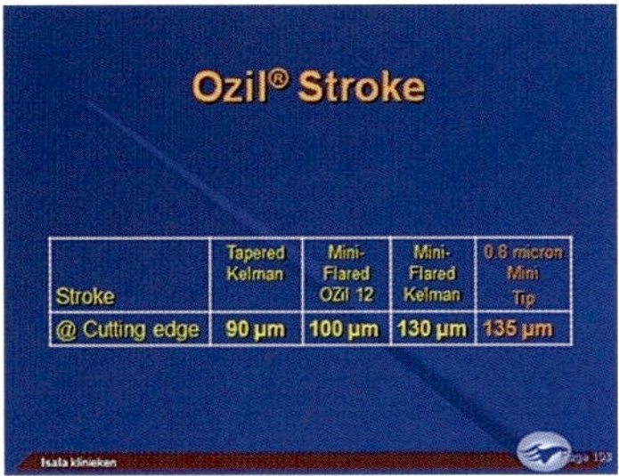

Fig. 35. Tip stroke.

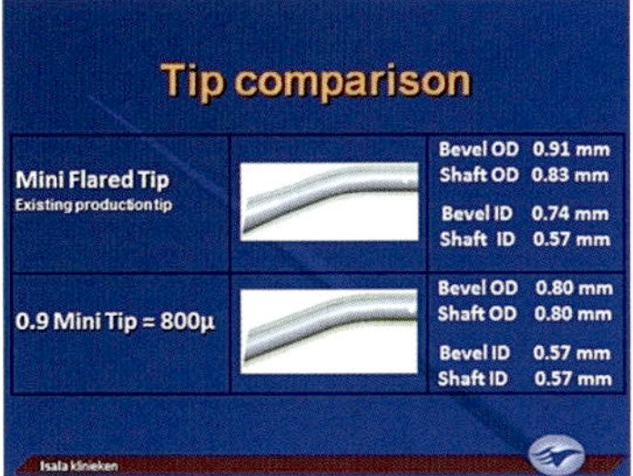

Fig. 36. Tip comparison.

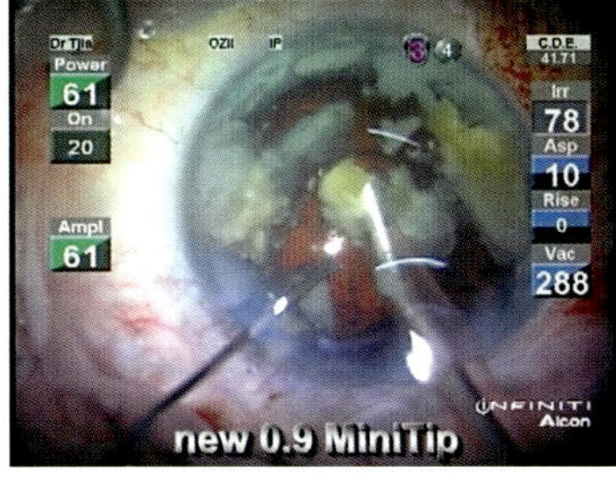

Fig. 37. 0.9 mini tip.

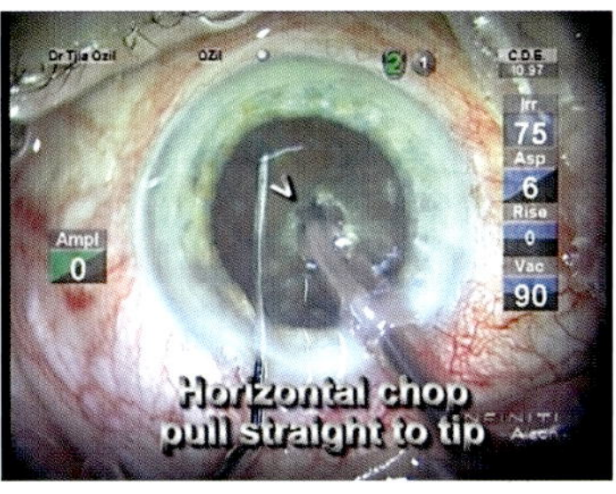

Fig. 38. Pull to tip.

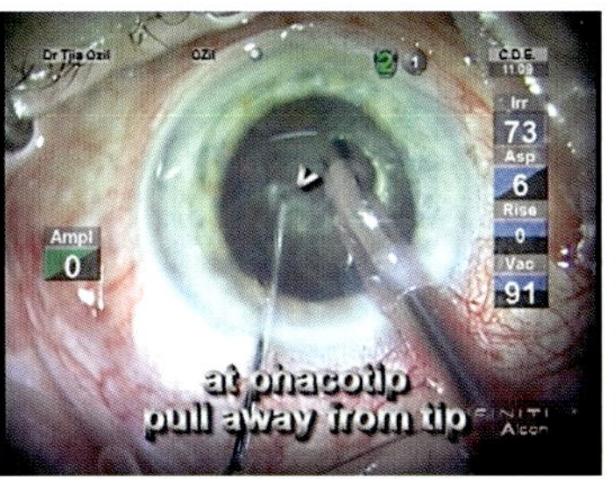

Fig. 39. Pull sideways.

Chop Techniques

Many chop techniques have been described. I shall only give a rough overview and provide a few personal comments. In general, chopping is performed to reduce the dissipated ultrasonic energy in the eye. It eliminates a great part of the energy of sculpting to divide the nucleus into smaller pieces. The chopping techniques are: (1) horizontal chop, with a dull tip end; (2) vertical chop, with a sharp tip end, and (3) prechop, proposed by Dr. Akahoshi, not discussed in this chapter.

Horizontal Chop

The basic principle of horizontal chop is drill the phacotip into the middle of the nucleus, just proximal to the very center. Then place the chopper underneath the rhexis edge in the periphery and move the chopper horizontally in a straight line towards the phacotip (fig. 38). A sideways splitting movement should only be performed when the chopper has reached the phacotip end (fig. 39). If a lateral movement is made in the mid-periphery, the nucleus risks to tilt which can lead to unwanted stress to zonules. With denser lens material, the leathery nucleus may not split

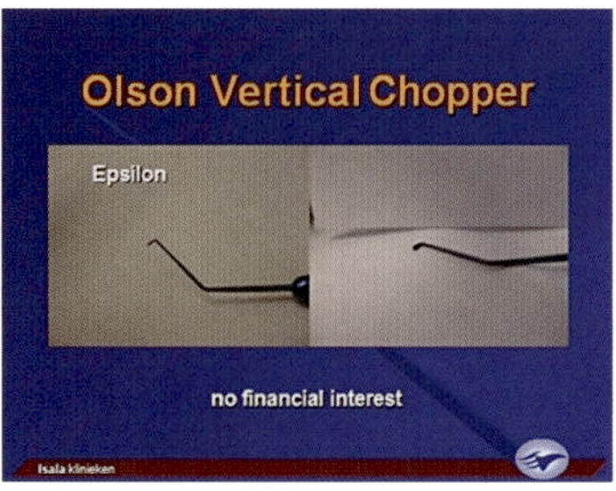

Fig. 40. Olson chopper.

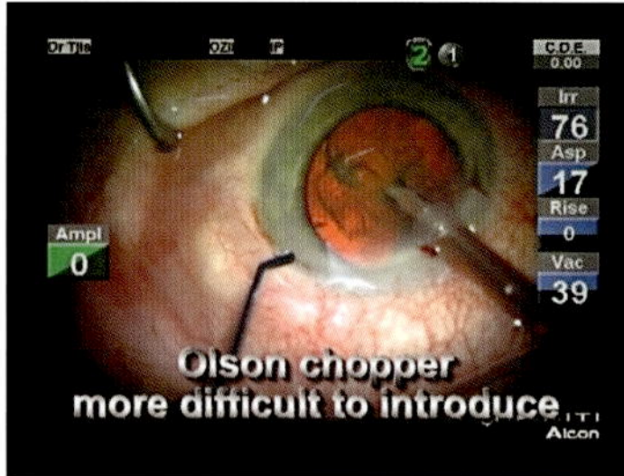

Fig. 41. Introduction.

completely. If so, one should take the phacotip back and drill in the nucleus at a deeper level and repeat the horizontal chop maneuver at the deeper level.

Vertical Chop

Vertical choppers are regarded to be suitable for more advanced surgeons. The traditional vertical chop instruments are sharp and pointed instruments which can easily split nuclei, but also potentially hazardous in the hands of an inexperienced surgeon. The surgical principle is that one should also drill the phacotip deep in the nucleus. The phacotip must have enough bare metal sticking out from the sleeve, in order to achieve a sufficient grip of the nucleus. The vertical chop instrument must then be placed just adjacent to the phacotip edge and pressed downwards, which creates a split in the nucleus.

Less experienced surgeons can consider an Olson modified vertical chopper, which has a bigger and round end. Although more difficult to introduce through the side port, which should be slightly larger, it is not so daunting for the surgeon, because of the lack of a sharp point (fig. 40–42).

Dense nuclei, with either the crack or chop technique, should be divided into more than 4 pieces. Dense nuclear quadrants can be difficult to emulsify, and during manipulation lead to the tilt of the quadrant and zonulolysis. A good guide-

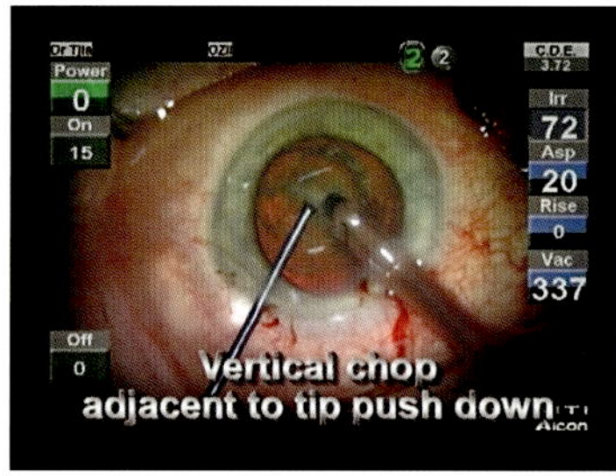

Fig. 42. Chop next to tip.

line is that grade 1 or 2 nuclei can be divided into 4 quadrants, but grade 3 into 6 pieces, and grade 4 into 8 or more.

Manual Chop

During the course, I show a few videos with a personal back-up technique, which I call 'manual chop'. If a regular cracking or chop technique fails to split the posterior nuclear plate, it can be extremely difficult and nerve-racking to complete the entire split in mostly very leathery and dense nuclei. There is normally no cortical layer underneath the nucleus to act as safety barrier between the phacotip/instruments and the posterior capsule. In such a case, I consider to inject some dispersive viscoelastic behind the nucleus to create some space for safer manipulation and subsequently continue with 2 slim instruments (e.g. a cracking and chop instrument) without any phacotip and fluidics in the eye. The anterior chamber can be filled with a viscoelastic substance to have a fully stabilized surgical field. The 2 instruments can then be utilized to manually split the remaining bridge between nuclear pieces. The absence of any fluid movement ensures the safety of the surgical manipulations. Less experienced surgeons can also use this as a backup technique. It only requires the moment of recognition that one should change surgical strategy to a very different but much safer technique.

Narrow Pupils and Synechiae

Narrow Pupil Surgical Strategies
There are several options to manage a small pupil case. Surgeon's skills and preferences will determine the level of surgeon's comfort and success of patient outcomes.

1 'Key hole surgery'; surgeon is comfortable with smaller pupil surgery and is very dependent on skills, not discussed here.
2 Multiple iridotomies; several small pupillotomies can be made with small scissors. Some bleeding usually occurs. This technique is not very widely used when more sophisticated devices are available to the surgeon.
3 Pupil stretching; either with a specially dedicated stretching device or just with two separate instruments, the pupil can be stretched in one direction. The instruments should be held in the periphery in opposite positions and held stable for a few seconds. The resulting oval pupil shape can be reformed to a round shape by simply injecting viscoelastic in the middle of the pupil. This eliminates multiple stretching maneuvers and limits trauma to the iris. This is a very cheap and still widely used technique and very often sufficient in

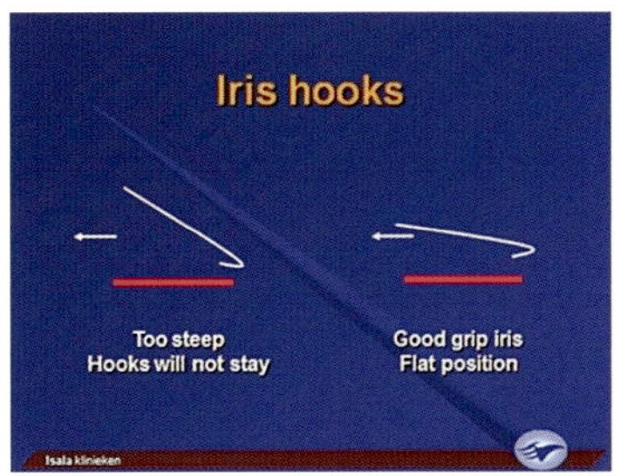

Fig. 43. Hook positioning.

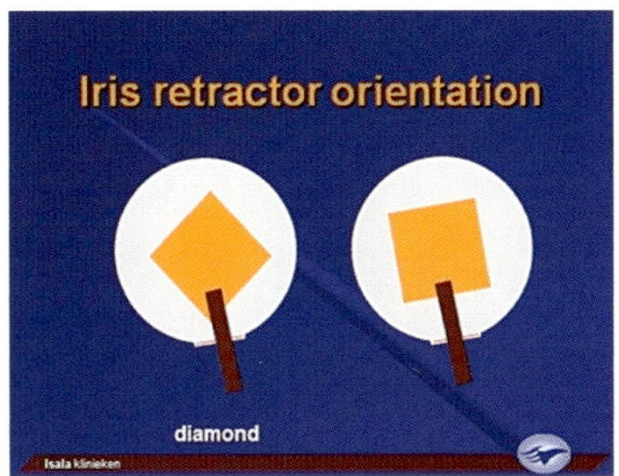

Fig. 44. Hook configuration.

the hands of reasonably experienced surgeons. It is not suitable for floppy iris cases.
4 Iris hooks; a more expensive solution, but very dependable and widely used. Four small incisions are created to introduce the iris hooks. The position incisions should be rather peripheral to obtain a flat angle of approach to the iris to facilitate capturing of the iris by the hooks (fig. 43). The orientation of the incisions near the main phacoincision is sometimes warranted in a way to obtain a diamond shape pupil, with one iris hook close to the main incision retracting the pupil away from the site where the phacotip enters the anterior chamber (fig. 44).

Pupil-stabilizing rings; the Malyugin ring is the most widely known and used, but there are

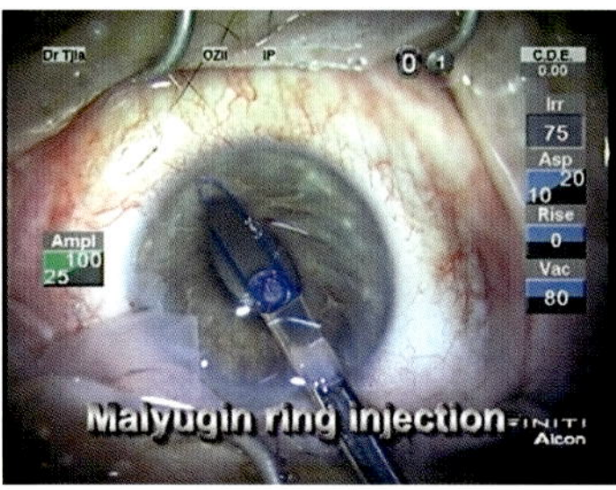

Fig. 45. Ring injection.

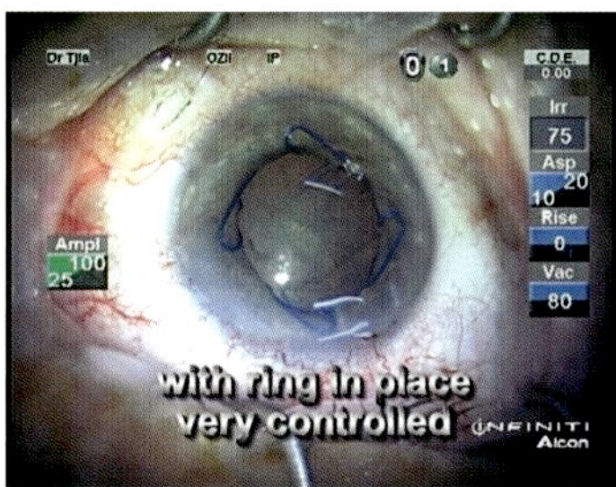

Fig. 46. Control.

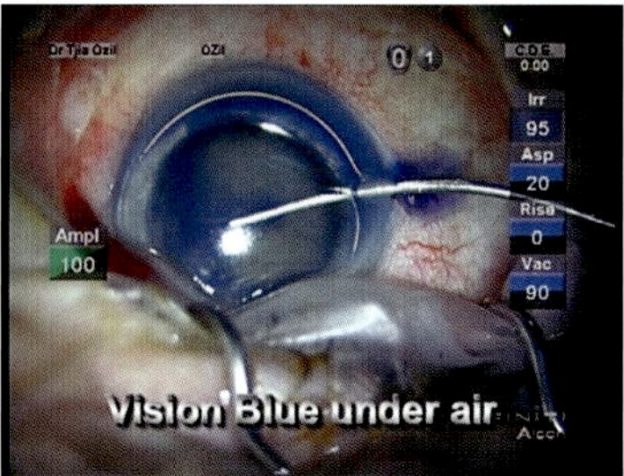

Fig. 47. Under air.

persive or viscoadaptive viscoelastic is mandatory to create space. It is important to work through very small incisions during capsulorhexis formation to prevent viscoelastic regressing from the anterior chamber, thereby reducing working space. A needle technique or microcapsulorhexis forceps for continuous curvilinear capsulorhexis (CCC) are both suitable for this situation.

other devices on the market. I have no personal experience other than with the Malyugin ring. This ring is an excellent pupil-stabilizing device, with a short learning curve (fig. 45). It requires learning a few small tips and tricks, which can be easily acquired through observing a few videos available on the internet (e.g. eyetube). Once installed in the eye, the Malyugin ring transforms extremely difficult and challenging small pupil cases into perfectly manageable cases (fig. 46).

If posterior synechiae are present, I personally prefer to dissect them by injecting a viscoelastic. This is the least traumatic technique to resolve synechiae. Sometimes, mechanical manipulation is still required. Fibrotic membranes can sometimes be peeled from the pupillary edge with capsulorhexis forceps.

In a very shallow anterior chamber case with possible anterior synechiae, injection with a dis-

Mature Cataracts

Mature cataracts share the lack of sufficient red reflex for creating a capsulorhexis easily. Staining of the anterior capsule with trypan blue transitions this hazardous situation into a very manageable one (fig. 48). Trypan blue can be injected into the anterior chamber directly, but I prefer to inject under air for better staining of the capsule (fig. 47). It is even possible to 'paintbrush' the capsule when the anterior chamber is already filled with viscoelastic (fig. 49).

The main question before starting surgery is whether the mature lens is swollen or not. A hypermature swollen lens needs to be decompressed as described below before any other manipulation. Another potential danger should be kept in mind when dealing with mature cataracts; capsules, and posterior capsules in particular are more fragile and very easy to rupture!

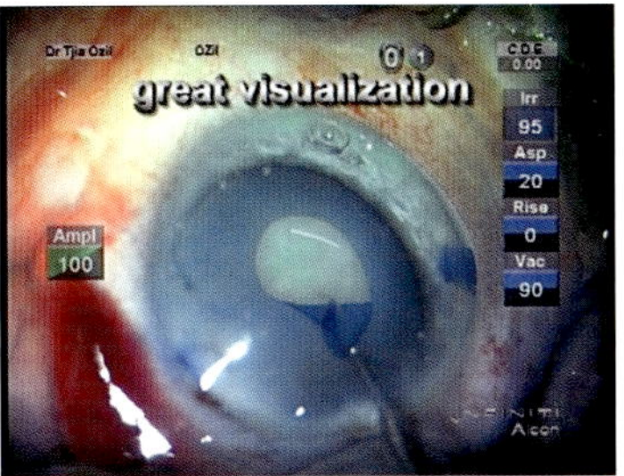

Fig. 48. Good visualization.

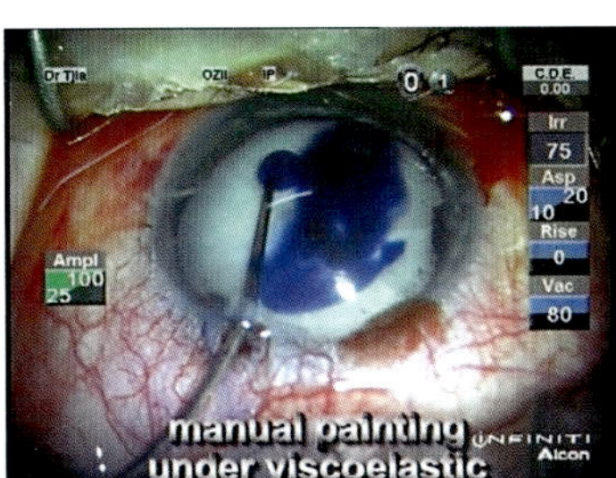

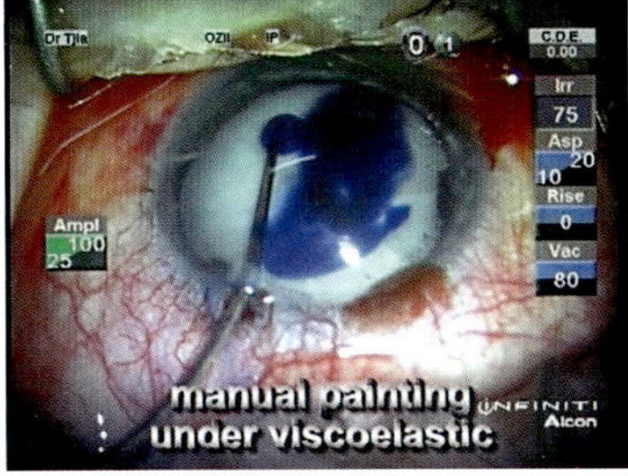

Fig. 49. Manual painting.

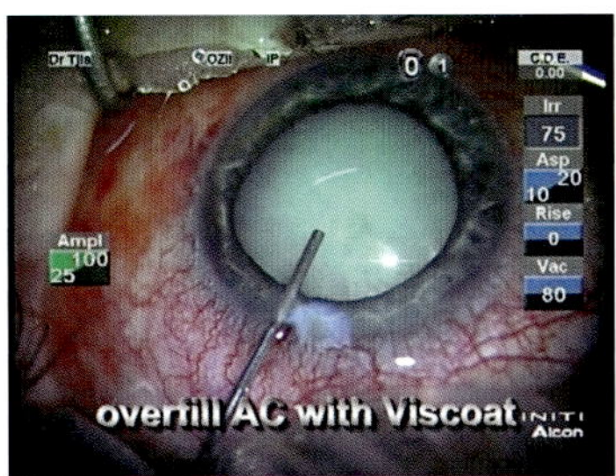

Fig. 50. Overfill AC.

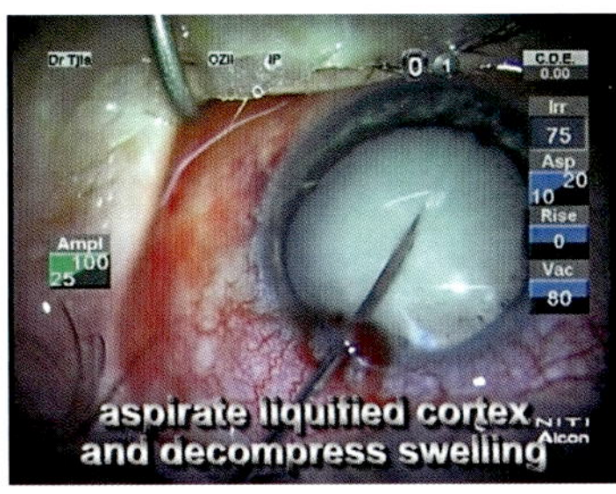

Fig. 51. Aspirate directly.

Hypermature White Intumescent Cataract

A hypermature white intumescent cataract can turn into a real nightmare for the cataract surgeon if the necessary precautions are not taken.

The hypermature cataract is characterized by a swelling of the lens and liquefying of lens material. The swollen content of the lens bag develops a higher intralenticular pressure with stretching of the lens capsule. When an intumescent hypermature cataract is punctured without any precaution, it can suddenly 'explode' with an instantaneous anterior capsule rupture extending into the zonules. This is very well known as the 'Argentinian Flag' sign; the clear white cataract zone between Vision Blue-dyed capsule mimics the Argentinian Flag. Upon suspicion of a swollen hyper mature cataract, the cataract surgeon should take the following precautions:

– Overfill the anterior chamber with viscoelastic to flatten the bulging anterior capsule and to exert counter-pressure to the swollen lens bag (fig. 50)
– Relieve the elevated capsular bag pressure by aspirating liquefied lens material whilst puncturing the lens with a sharp 27-gauge needle. The needle should be introduced into the anterior chamber through a very small side port incision to avoid viscoelastic leakage and to maintain the high pressure in the anterior chamber (fig. 51)
– Once the hypermature cataract is decompressed, spontaneous explosive extension of the anterior capsulotomy will no longer occur (fig. 52). The anterior capsule can then be safely dyed with Vision Blue by 'painting' the capsule underneath the

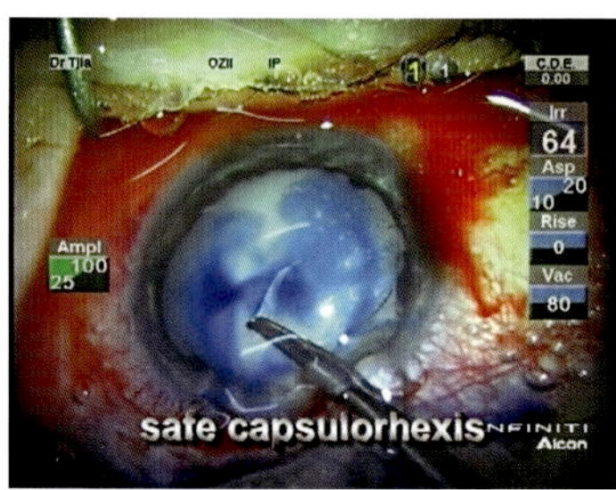

Fig. 52. Safe rhexis.

viscoelastic substance. After successful capsulorhexis formation, phacoemulsification should be relatively normal. The posterior capsule can be weaker than normal, but if handled with care, the case can be handled properly

Intraoperative Floppy Iris Syndrome

Since 2005, intraoperative floppy iris syndrome (IFIS) has become a very well-known complicated cataract case. Chang and Campbell described the condition in great detail. It is not my intention to write another overview article on IFIS. There have been many very good articles published in recent years. Still, I do want to provide a practical guideline for an unexpected floppy iris case.

Let us suppose that you are suddenly confronted with an iris which starts to billow during hydrodissection. And upon starting ultrasound phacoprocedure, iris starts to move around in a typical 'floppy' way. There are 4 different strategies which can help to manage such an IFIS case. They all aim at stabilization of the iris diaphragm:

Pharmacological Compounds
Intracameral epinephrine has been proven to be helpful in stabilizing the iris. Dr. Shugar started using the combination of lidocaine and epinephrine (epi-Shugarcaine). In my own setting, I use a

minim of unpreserved phenylephrine 2.5% which contains 0.4 ml, and dilute this with balanced salt solution to a total volume of 1 ml.

Mechanical Devices
Some surgeons rapidly choose to stabilize the iris mechanically. In most operating theatres, iris hooks will be available for this purpose. I prefer the Malyugin ring to stabilize the iris in a severe floppy iris case.

Viscoelastic Substances
Dispersive viscoelastics can be very helpful to dampen the iris mobility. Injecting sufficient amounts of a dispersive viscoelastic both on top as well as underneath the iris can assist in reducing the tendency of the iris to move along with the fluid streams in the eye.

Fluid Dynamics
Personally, I have been able to manage very floppy iris cases with a combination of a suitable viscoelastic and very low flow fluid dynamics settings.

The key issue is that a floppy iris will move along with the fluid streams in the eye. High fluid streams in the anterior chamber will drag a floppy iris along to wherever the fluid is going to, phacotip or leaking incisions. It is therefore essential to follow a strategy which minimizes the fluid movements in the eye.

I will try to explain this strategy step by step:
1 Eliminate leak flow through the main incision; make sure that the phacosleeve closes off the main incision completely. One should even consider creating a new incision if necessary.
2 Minimize leak flow through the side port. If the initial side port is too large, one should consider making a new one, as small as possible (fig. 53, 54).
3 Minimize the infusion pressure by lowering the bottle as low as 40–50 cm. (A high infusion pressure increases leak flow.)

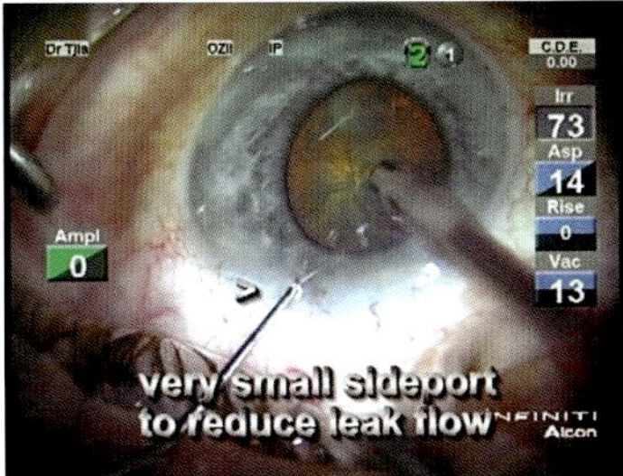

Fig. 53. Small sideport.

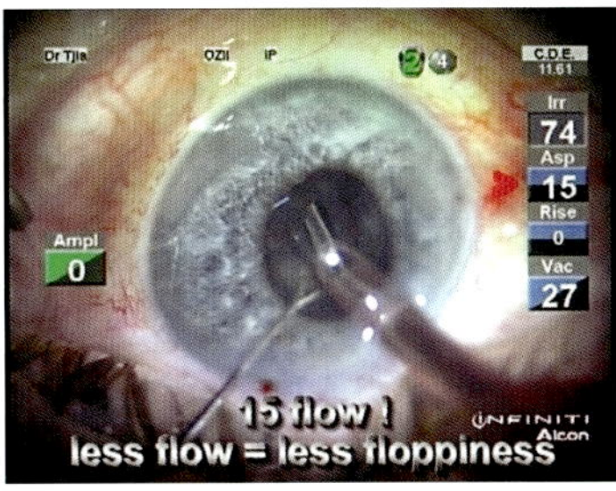

Fig. 55. Less floppy.

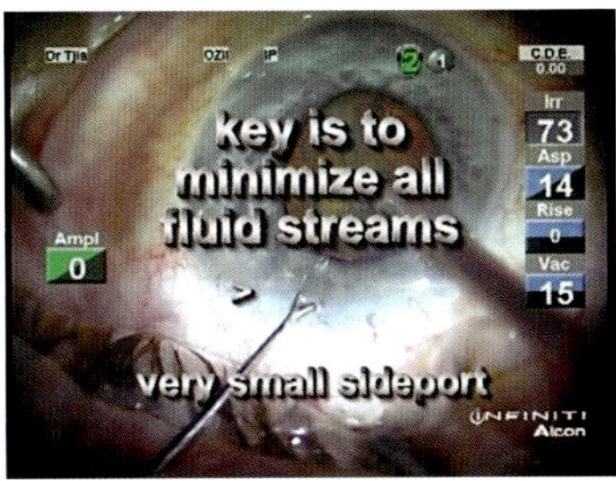

Fig. 54. Low leak flow.

4   Reduce aspiration flow settings to very low levels (12–15 ml/min; fig. 55).
5   Minimize aspiration flow by maintaining occlusion as much as possible. This is facilitated by torsional ultrasound because of the minimal intrinsic repulsion. With longitudinal ultrasound, one can reduce repulsion by lowering ultrasound on-time (duty cycle).
6   Reduce surge flow by using moderate vacuum levels. A sudden high surge flow on occlusion break can easily catch a floppy iris into the phacotip.
7   Inject dispersive or viscoadaptive viscoelastic substance around the entire iris, not only on top of the iris, but also some underneath the iris circumferentially. With the recommended aspiration flow levels, the viscoelastic will remain in place and will prevent the iris from moving with the (low) fluid streams in the anterior chamber.

I use Viscoat (Alcon Laboratories) to stabilize the iris. I prefer a lower molecular weight viscoelastic such as Viscoat because it does not cause very high pressure spikes postoperatively. It is very likely to leave some viscoelastic in the eye in a floppy iris case.

With this combined, dispersive viscoelastic 'wrap around the iris' + very low fluidics strategy and torsional ultrasound, I have been able to manage all floppy iris cases very safely. I recommend a 'very low flow 'setting for specific cases such as IFIS.

I present 3 pictures of a floppy iris case: 2 min, 38 s, 18 frames (fig. 56), 2 min, 38 s, 21 frames (fig. 57), and 2 min, 39 s, 2 frames (fig. 58), depicting the floppiness of an iris within half a second. The aspiration flow setting in this case was 25 ml/min. Such an aspiration flow setting will aspirate the viscoelastic to some degree and will not prevent the iris from being floppy.

I switched to the proposed very low flow strategy after this case and have not been able to produce such a nice series of floppy iris pictures any more.

Weak Zonules

If an eye has not shown any signs or symptoms of suspected weak zonules preoperatively, this does not preclude the possibility of weak zonules during the procedure.

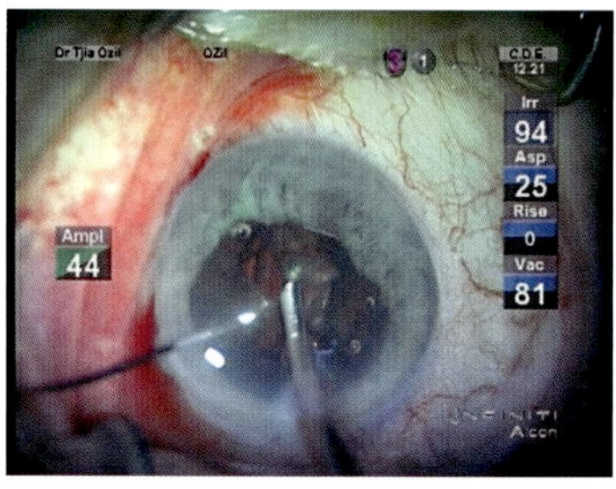

Fig. 56. Very floppy.

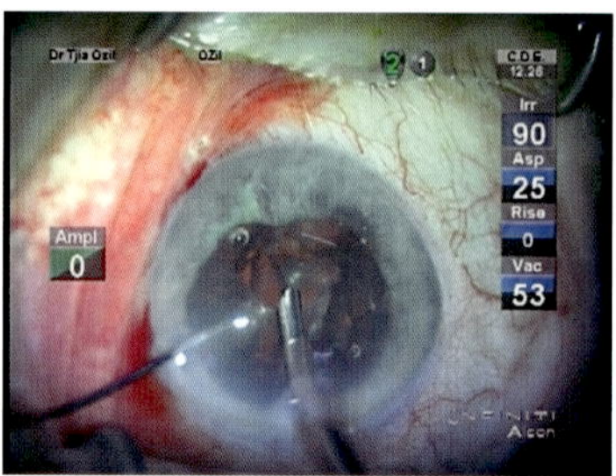

Fig. 58. Floppy iris case.

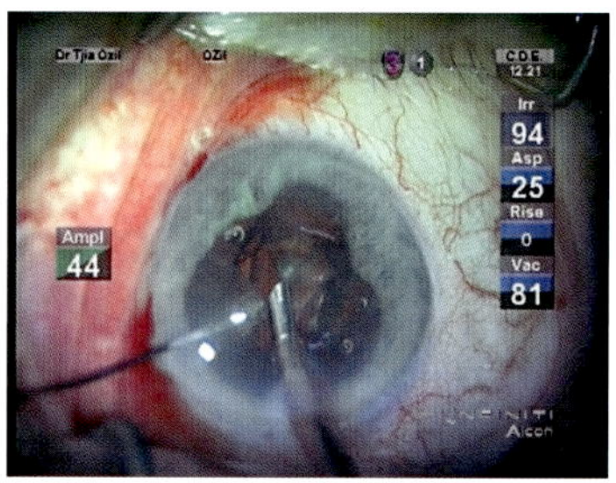

Fig. 57. Worm like movement.

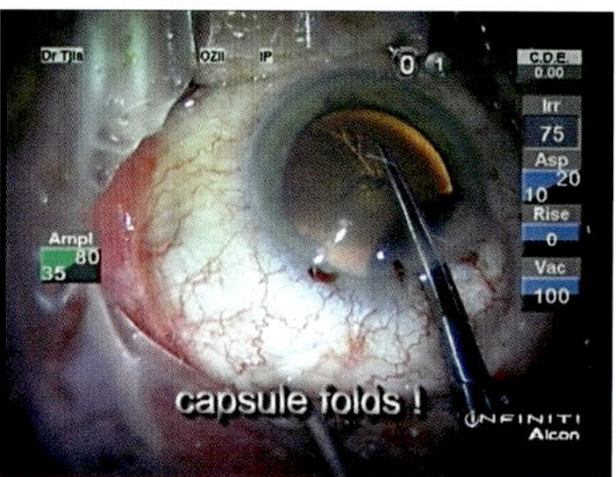

Fig. 59. Warning sign.

The warning sign of weak zonules is the occurrence of capsule folds during capsulorhexis formation (fig. 59). One has to be vigilant to this very important warning sign and initiate a very specific 'weak zonules' strategy immediately. The main principle is to reduce the stress to the zonules as much as possible. The following measures should be carried out with great caution:

1 Create a very large capsulorhexis. This reduces the mechanical impact of any manipulation in the eye to the zonules (fig. 60).
2 Perform very careful hydrodissection in multiple positions circumferentially and avoid early rotation attempts.
3 If hydrodissection is complete, bimanual rotation around the central axis of the lens is highly preferable to minimize stress to the zonules.
4 Sculpting should be performed at a slow pace with sufficient ultrasound energy to avoid 'pushing' of the lens. If the nucleus is pushed forward, there will be inadvertent traction on the zonules. The groove should be made sufficiently wide to avoid pushing of the nucleus by the sleeve (fig. 61).
5 Nucleus disassembly should be done in multiple and smaller pieces than usual. Subsequent manipulation and emulsification of fragments will cause less stress to the zonules. With greater density of nucleus, one should increase the number of cracks/chops even more.
6 Avoid the use of regular, nonsutured, tension rings in general zonule weakness cases. A significant number of complete late-onset total IOL/capsule dislocations have been reported.

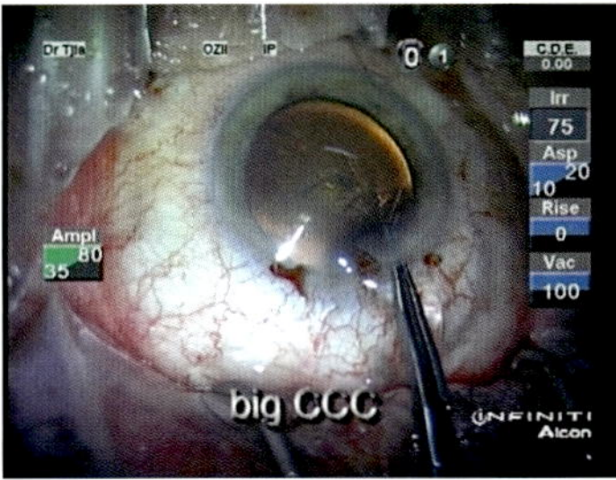

Fig. 60. Large CCC.

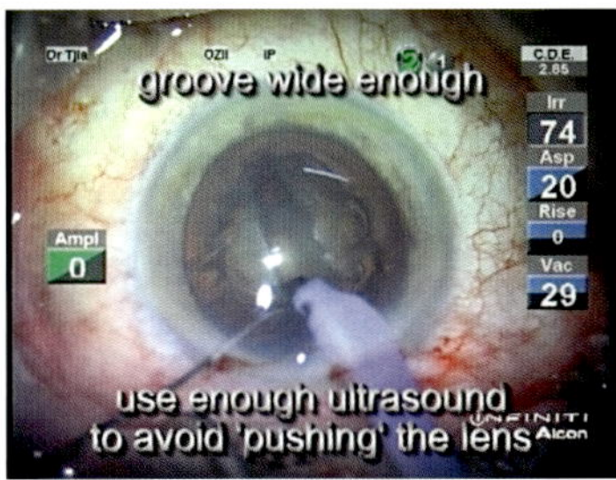

Fig. 61. Wider groove.

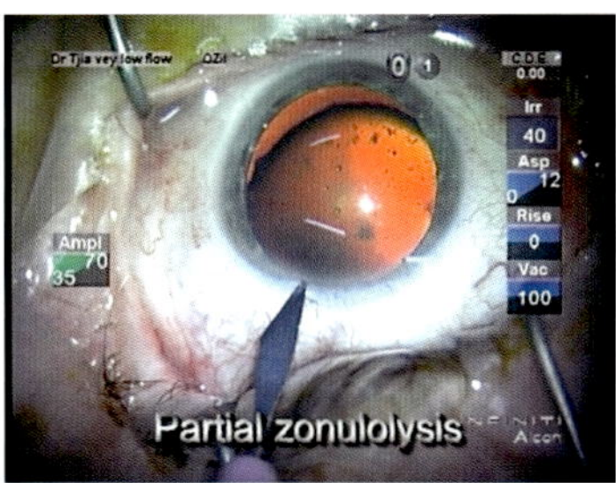

Fig. 62. Zonulolysis.

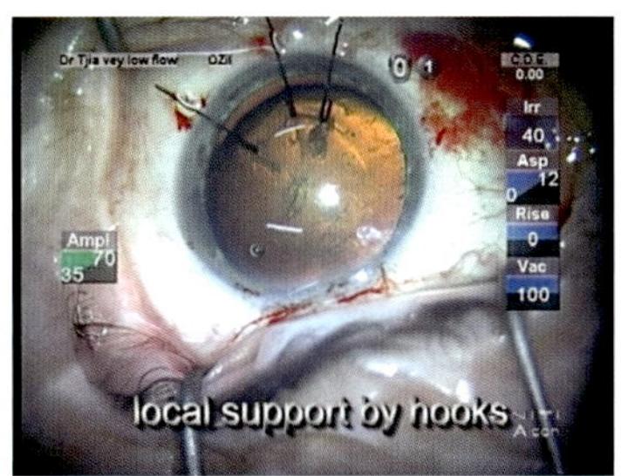

Fig. 63. Hook support.

7 Implement a lower fluidics settings strategy to reduce the fluid turbulence which could negatively impact the zonules' integrity.

Zonulolysis

With a preexisting zonular defect, one has to distinguish a local (e.g. a posttraumatic) defect from a generalized weak zonules case with a symptomatic area of zonulolysis. A partial defect, which is not too large and with otherwise healthy zonules, can be managed by placing a regular tension ring (fig. 62, 63, 65). Potential presence of vitreous through the defect should be detected at an early stage and removed prior to further action. (anterior vitrectomy, see other topics).

A very low fluidics strategy is recommended to avoid high pressure changes and turbulence, all of

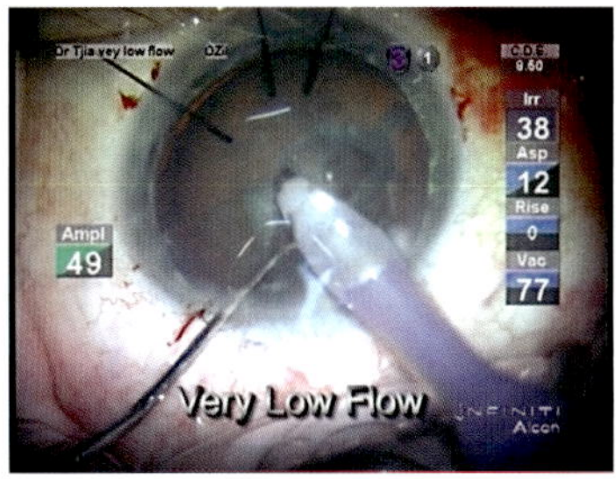

Fig. 64. Very low flow.

which can disturb the brittle equilibrium of such a complicated case (fig. 64).

A generalized zonular weakness case with partial lysis is probably amongst the most challenging cases for a cataract surgeon. The treatment of such a very complicated case is probably beyond the scope of this chapter, and referral of such a

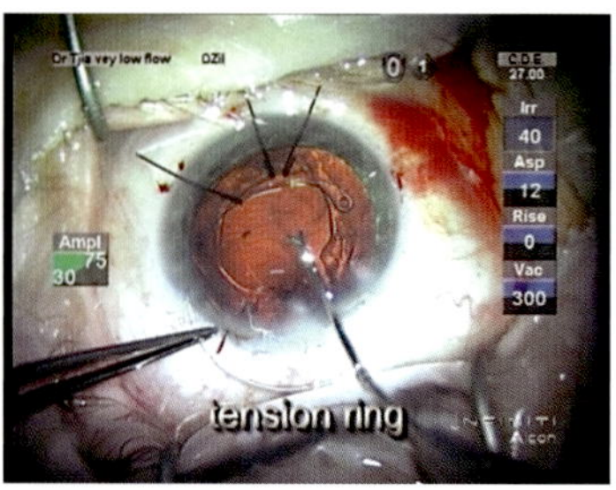

Fig. 65. Tension ring.

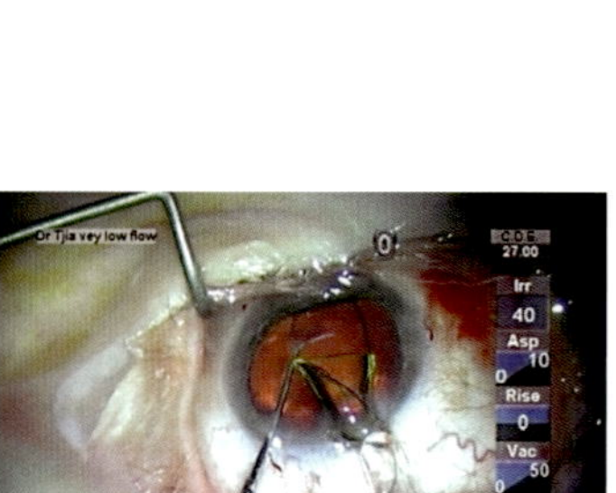

Fig. 66. Sulcus support iol.

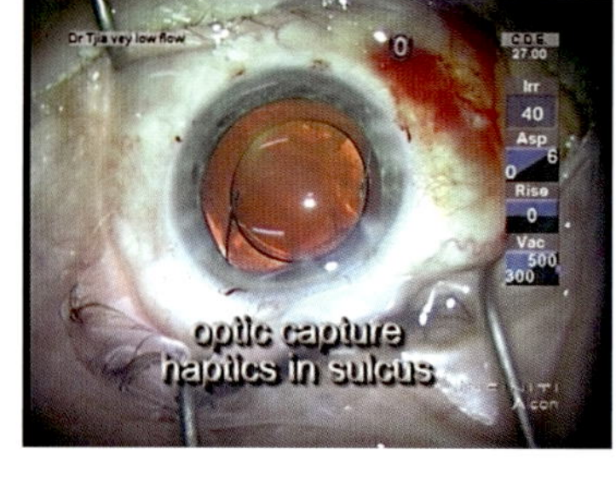

Fig. 67. Optic capture.

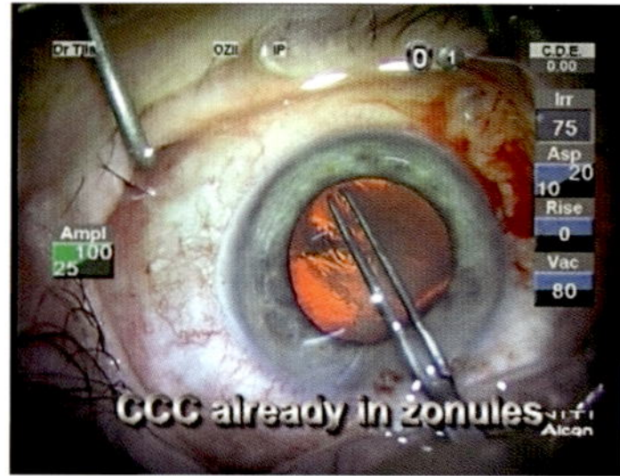

Fig. 68. CCC tear out.

case to an experienced colleague should be considered. Innovative devices, such as capsule hooks, Cionni modified tension rings, Ahmed segments or Assia capsule anchor can be utilized to manage such a case successfully, but all devices involve a learning curve and higher complication rates.

In any weak zonules/zonulolysis case where there might be insufficient long-term stability of the lens capsule/zonules complex, one should consider implanting a 3-piece sulcus-fixated IOL with posterior angulation (fig. 66, 67).

Capsule Rupture

Anterior Capsule Rupture
An anterior capsule rupture which does not extend into the zonules can be salvaged by simply pulling the loose end of the torn flap back to the center to create a continuous capsulorhexis.

When the tear is already in the zonule region (fig. 68), one should practice the 'pull back' technique. The capsule needs to be caught with capsulorhexis forceps very near to the end of the tear. The forceps should then be directed in a 'backward' direction; not forward, not towards the center, but almost in the opposite direction of the normal capsulorhexis creation (fig. 69). Once liberated from the zonules, the capsulorhexis can be finished in a regular fashion (fig. 70).

Posterior Capsule Rupture
Whenever a posterior capsule rupture is suspected, the most important thing to remember is: do not follow your impulse to retract everything

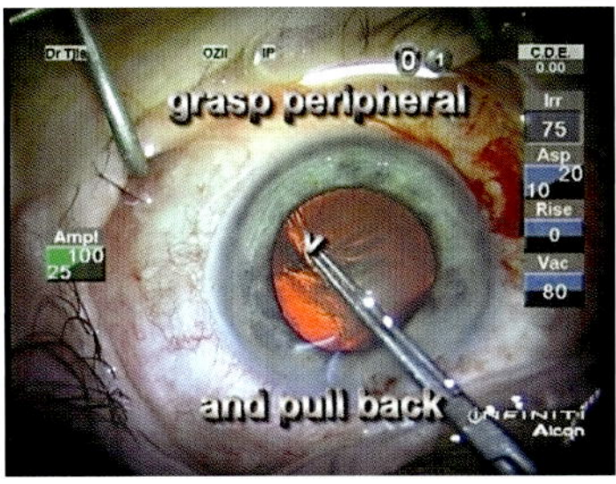

Fig. 69. Pull back maneuver.

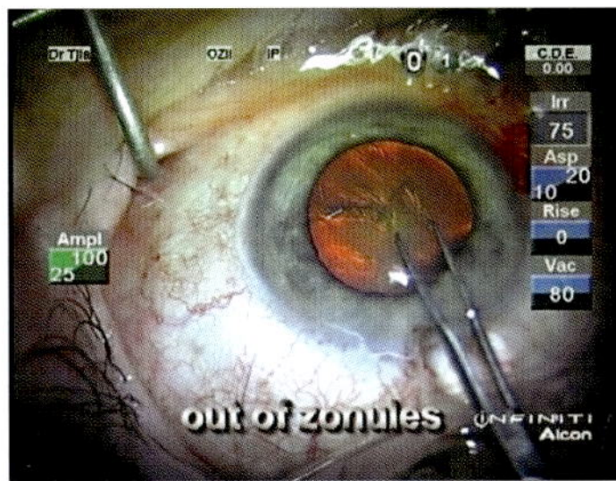

Fig. 70. CCC rescued.

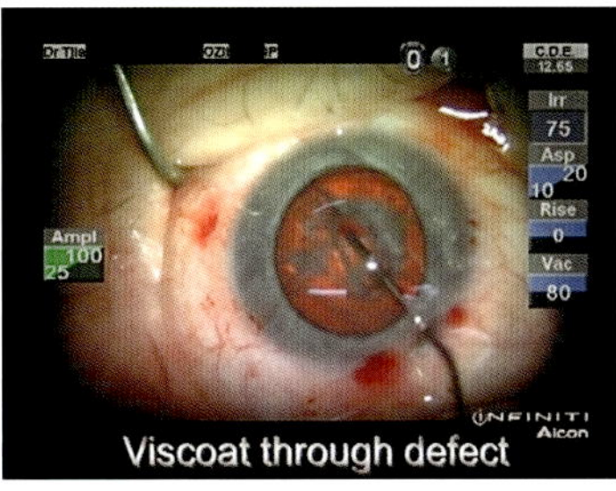

Fig. 71. Viscoat through defect.

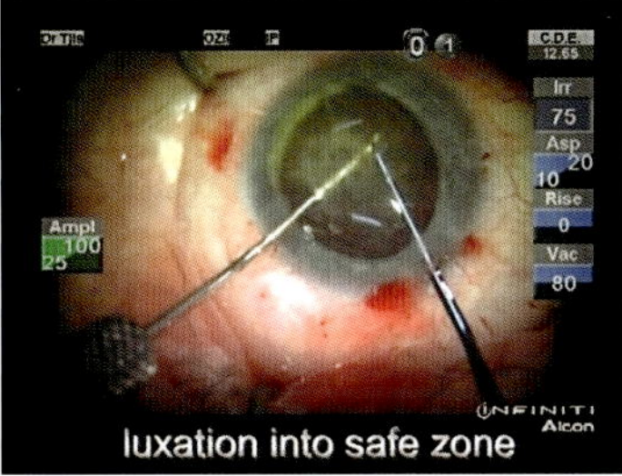

Fig. 72. Safe zone.

from the eye! The sudden change of volume in the anterior chamber can lead to direct extension of the posterior capsule tear and displacement of nuclear fragments to the posterior segment. The dogma to follow is: 'Hold the phacotip still in the eye!' The second instrument can be carefully withdrawn from the eye (not much change in volume), and inject any viscoelastic available in the area of the suspected rupture to stabilize lens fragments and prevent them from falling back. If this has been executed successfully, one can retract the phacotip and take a deep breath of relief. Then a very important decision has to be taken – consult a colleague or continue by yourself. If the decision is to proceed, my recommended measures are:

1 Lower bottle height, aspiration flow and vacuum; have a dedicated low flow program preset.

2 Inject a dispersive viscoelastic through the posterior capsule rupture to install a 'dispersive viscoshield barrier' (fig. 71).

3 If vitreous is suspected to be already present in the anterior chamber, inject diluted (approx. 10×) triamcinolone in the anterior chamber to 'stain' vitreous. If vitreous is detected, this should be removed by careful bimanual low-flow anterior vitrectomy to prevent traction to the retina.

4 Reinstall the viscoshield barrier as often as needed to prevent nuclear fragments falling to the posterior segment. I personally inject profuse amounts of dispersive viscoelastic to make sure that nothing can pass this barrier to the vitreous.

5 The nuclear pieces need to be elevated manually to a safe position far enough from the capsule rupture (fig. 72).

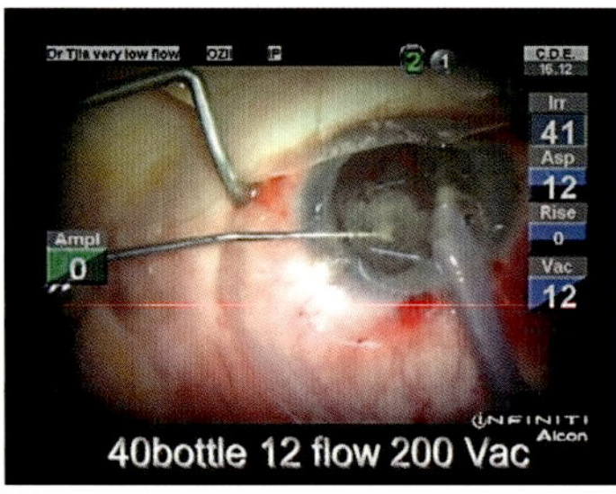

Fig. 73. Very low flow.

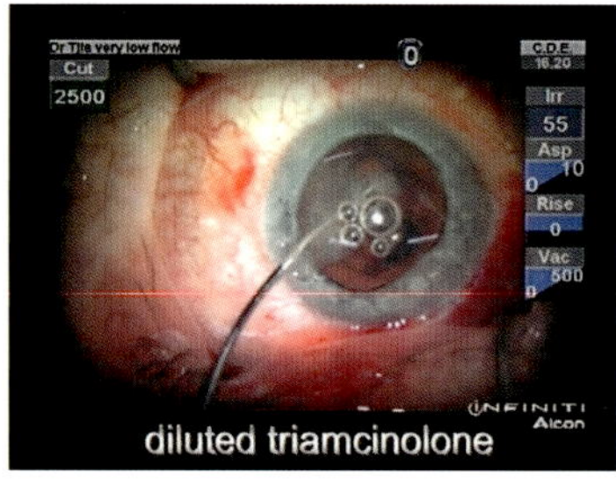

Fig. 74. Triamcinolone.

6   Emulsification of these nuclear fragments should be performed at a very low flow setting to limit the removal of the viscoelastic barrier as much as possible (fig. 73). The vacuum should be very moderate to reduce the occlusion break surge response; my personal settings for the Infiniti machine (which can be translated into comparable settings for other machines) are 40 cm bottle, 12 ml/min flow, 200 mm Hg vacuum. Torsional ultrasound settings can remain normal because of the lack of repulsion. With longitudinal ultrasound, power settings should be limited and duty cycle decreased to reduce the phenomenon of repulsion as much as possible.

7   After completion of nucleus removal (with repeated dispersive viscoelastic injection if necessary), bimanual anterior vitrectomy through 2 side ports can be initiated. Make sure that the side ports do not allow significant leak flow, as any flow might drag along vitreous with traction to the retina as a result. A bimanual system with separated irrigation and vitrectomy/aspiration is mandatory (fig. 75).

8   Inject diluted triamcinolone to detect any remaining vitreous (fig. 74), and remove by vitrectomy if applicable.

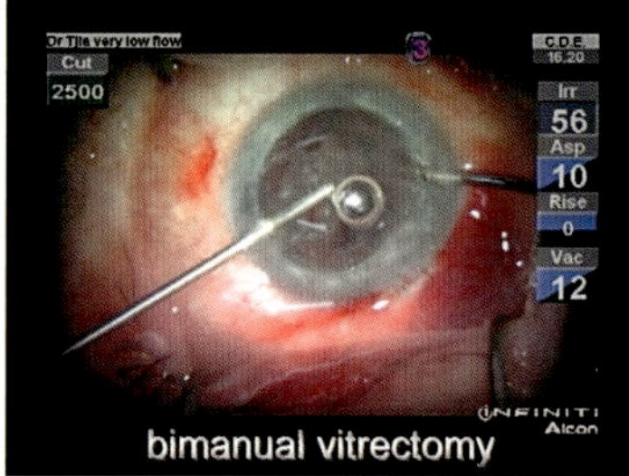

Fig. 75. Closed system.

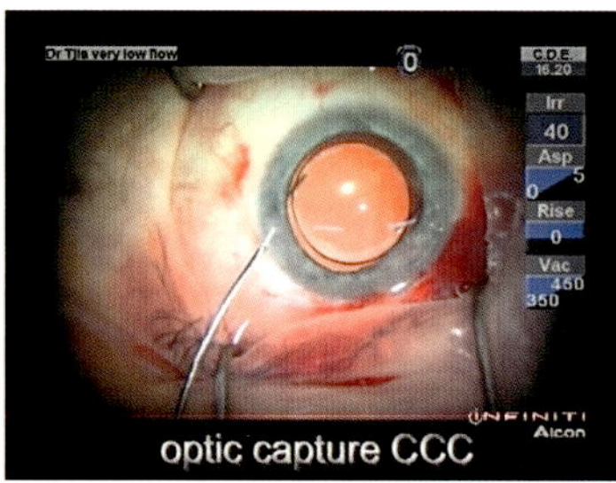

Fig. 76. Optic capture.

9   After removal of all vitreous, bimanual irrigation/aspiration of residual cortex through the same side ports follows. A very low aspiration flow of 5 ml/min is preferred to minimize the risk of vitreous aspiration.

10 If the CCC is intact, a sulcus-fixated 3-piece IOL implantation is the most convenient solution. Optic capture through the CCC is favorable for IOL stabilization and sequestration of the posterior segment (fig. 76). The IOL can be implanted with an injector or forceps, depending on the surgeon's experience and instrumentation availability. A regular nonangulated single-piece IOL is not designed for sulcus fixation. The sharp edges of the lens can easily come into contact with the back side of the iris, which can lead to potential pigment loss and inflammation.

Khiun Tjia
Isala Clinics
Groot Wezenland 20
8011JW Zwolle (The Netherlands)
E-Mail kftjia@gmail.com

Güell JL (ed): Cataract. ESASO Course Series. Basel, Karger, 2013, vol 3, pp 26–37
DOI: 10.1159/000350900

Multifocal and Accommodative Intraocular Lenses

Roberto Bellucci

Ophthalmic Unit, Department of Neurosciences, Hospital and University of Verona, Verona, Italy

Abstract

Multifocal intraocular lenses (IOLs) have at least two dioptric powers, providing at least two different foci on the same axis. They generate at least two superimposed images of each observed object. Image confusion is reduced by distant power asphericity, near power apodization, and different distance-near light distribution. At the moment, diffractive multifocal IOLs are the most successful. Results show good distance and near visual acuity, reduced contrast sensitivity and good patient satisfaction. Halos and glare are the most frequently reported problems, occasionally causing IOL explantation. Pseudoaccommodative IOLs are monofocal IOLs that change power with accommodation, usually by forward optic displacement. Their ability to provide good distance and near vision has not been universally confirmed in clinical practice.

For many years, attempts have been made to solve the main problem of pseudophakia – the loss of accommodation. Some of the approaches are based on modifications of the intraocular lens (IOL) in order to provide multifocality or pseudoaccommodation.

Multifocal Intraocular Lenses

The first multifocal IOL gaining some diffusion in clinical practice had diffractive optics, with the bifocal add designed as a Fresnel lens on the posterior optic surface [1]. Bifocal refractive IOLs with different optical zones devoted to distance and to near vision appeared at the same time [2]. Despite the reported good results, multifocal IOL never gained wide acceptance. The difficulties in astigmatism control with PMMA lenses, the visual problems reported by some patients and cost were among the possible causes.

Diffractive multifocal IOLs use Fresnel's principle. One of the lens surfaces hosts a series of visible concentric rings that testify the presence of the second dioptric power, the base power plus the near add (fig. 1). This type of surface causes diffraction of part of the refracted light onto a second focus, corresponding to the second lens power. For each ring, the second dioptric power determines the gradient of the slope. The maximum amount of diffracted light is 50%, a figure that can be reduced by decreasing the height and/ or the number of the rings.

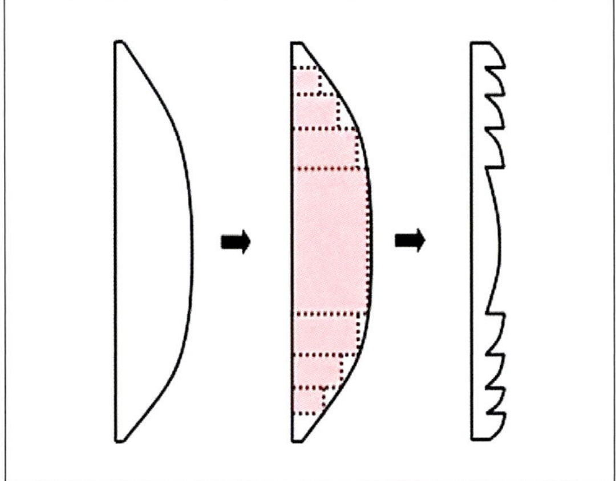

Fig. 1. Fresnel's principle to reduce lens thickness is applied to diffractive multifocal IOLs.

Refractive multifocal IOLs alternate distance power and near power concentrically (fig. 2). Usually, the central part of the lens is dedicated to distant vision, and the first annular part to near vision. Recently, zonal multifocal IOLs have been proposed, with a partial annular part for near vision.

The Problem of Multifocality: Image Confusion
Regardless of the adopted principle, diffractive or refractive, multifocal IOLs have two or more co-axial optical foci. This means the presence of at least two coaxial dioptric powers, usually separated by a 3.0- to 4.0-dpt interval to provide a 2.5- to 3.0-dpt interval at the spectacle plane. On the retina, the two dioptric powers will produce two superimposed images of any observed object [3]. Under the best conditions, one image will be in sharp focus, and the other image will be blurred by a 3-dpt defocus aberration (fig. 3). For example, a black dot on white paper will appear surrounded by a grey halo, and a black line by a narrow grey ribbon. This is the optical reason for the reduction in modulation transfer function (MTF) observed with multifocal IOLs [4], unfortunately a reduction strictly connected to the presence of coaxial different powers. This lower optical quality as compared with monofocal IOLs emerges as lower contrast sensitivity in implanted patients [3].

Approaches to Reduce Confusion and Improve Contrast Sensitivity
To overcome this problem, optical engineers developed several solutions, with the purpose of improving light transmission and reducing image confusion.

Light transmission can be improved by reducing the amount of dispersed light. In diffractive lenses, this is obtained by improving the ring edge profile design to minimize glare and halos [5]. The Acri.LISA (Carl Zeiss, Oberocken, Germany) and the SeeLens MF (Hanita Lenses, Hanita, Israel) are two examples of this approach (fig. 4). In refractive lenses, this is obtained by careful control of transition zones, as implemented in the ReZoom IOL [6] (AMO, Santa Ana, Calif., USA; fig. 5).

Image confusion can be reduced in several ways. The two foci should be as sharp as possible, and any depth of focus should be avoided. Therefore, we should employ only aspheric optics, possibly correcting for the corneal spherical aberration. At the moment, all the multifocal IOLs have aspheric profiles, with the Tecnis MF (AMO) being the prototype of this approach [7] (fig. 6). In addition, the amount of light directed onto the two foci can be different, thus privileging distance or near vision. Distance-dominant multifocal IOLs provide higher contrast sensitivity for distance focus, and lower contrast sensitivity for near focus, while the contrary happens with near-dominant multifocal IOLs [8].

A further approach is to get some help from the pupil, driving different amounts of light on the different foci depending on pupil dilation and trying to adapt to the visual task. This is obtained by apodization, i.e. by designing diffractive rings of decreasing height with increasing eccentricity, and only in the central part of the IOL surface (fig. 7). By apodization, according to pupil size,

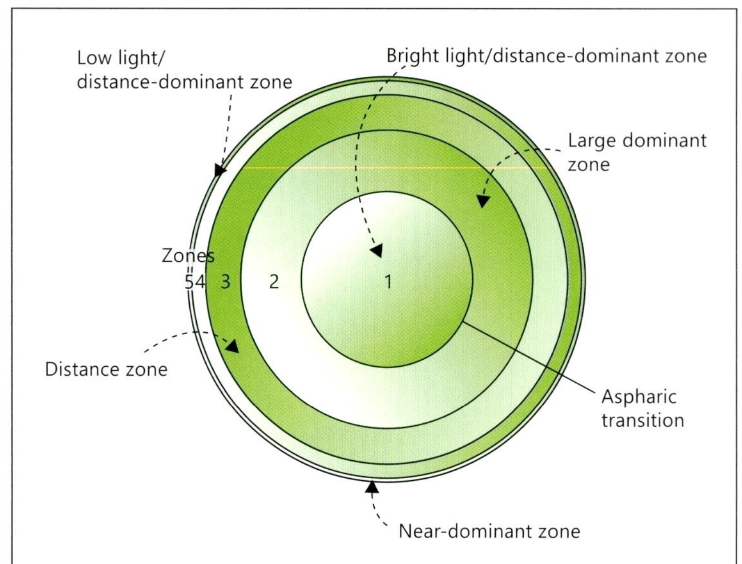

Fig. 2. Zonal refractive multifocality means concentric zones of different power.

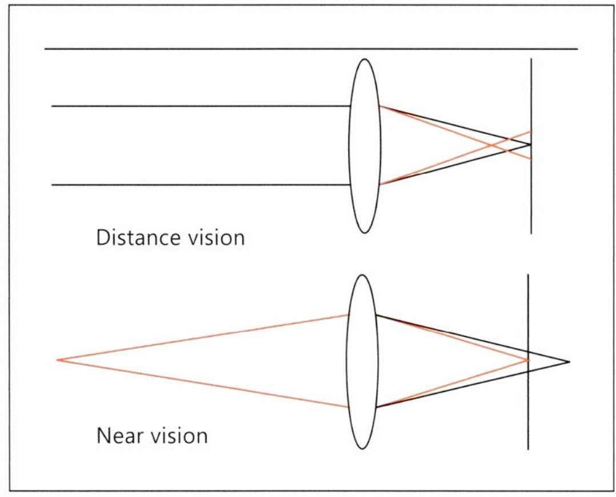

Fig. 3. Multifocality means two optical powers/foci. They produce two images of the observed object. The two images confound each other.

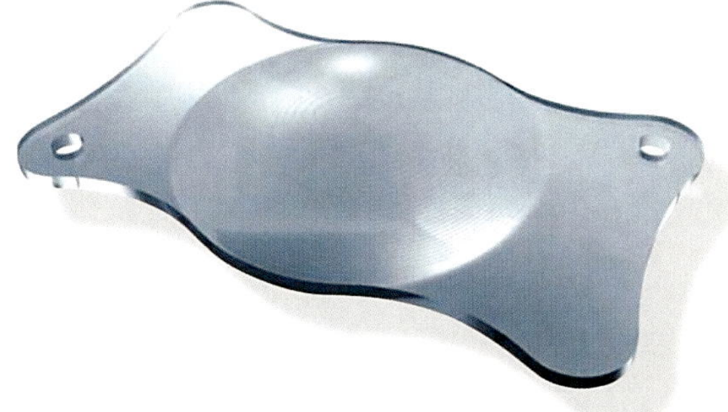

Fig. 4. Acri.LISA IOL (Zeiss, Jena, Germany) with 60:40 distant/near light distribution.

40–90% of the refracted light is directed onto the far focus (fig. 8). The well-known hydrophobic acrylic Acrysof ReSTOR (Alcon, Forth Worth, Tex., USA) and the hydrophilic acrylic SeeLens MF (Hanita Lenses) are two examples of this approach that claims to reduce glare during night driving [9–11].

By alternating rings of different slopes, additional powers can be implemented onto a lens surface; this can be used to improve poor intermediate vision, one of the major drawbacks of multifocal IOLs. For optical reasons, the amount of the intermediate add should be half as the near add. The FINE Vision IOL (PhysIOL, Liege, Belgium) provides 2 apodized dioptric adds (+1.75 and +3.50 dpt at the IOL plane), and showed excellent results in the first clinical trials (fig. 9). From an optical point of view, this trifo-

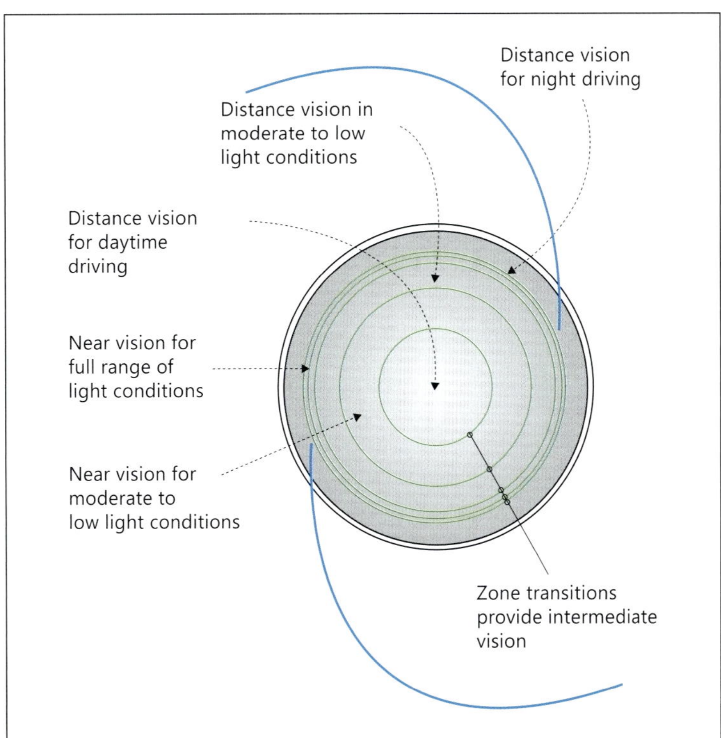

Fig. 5. ReZoom refractive multifocal IOL (AMO).

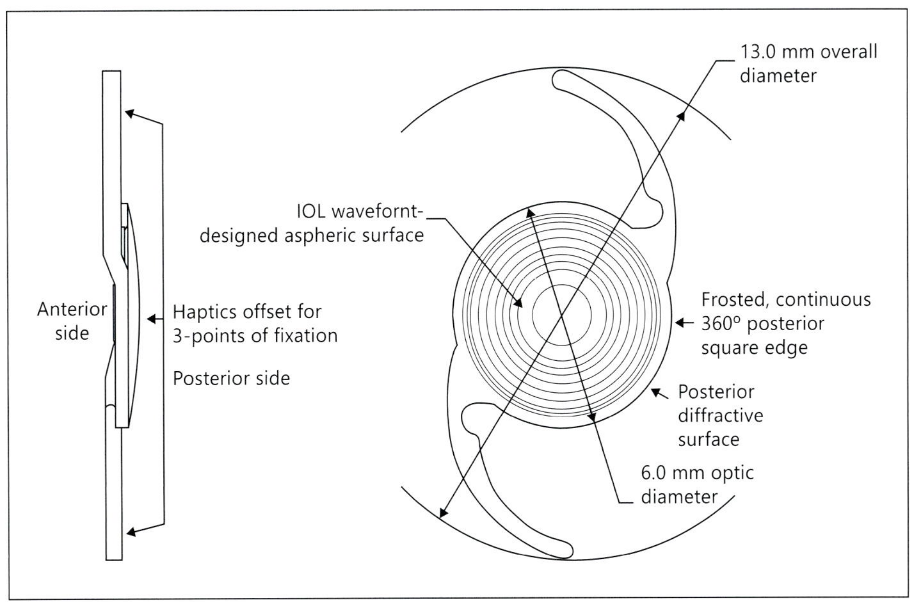

Fig. 6. Tecnis diffractive multifocal IOL with 50:50 light distribution (AMO).

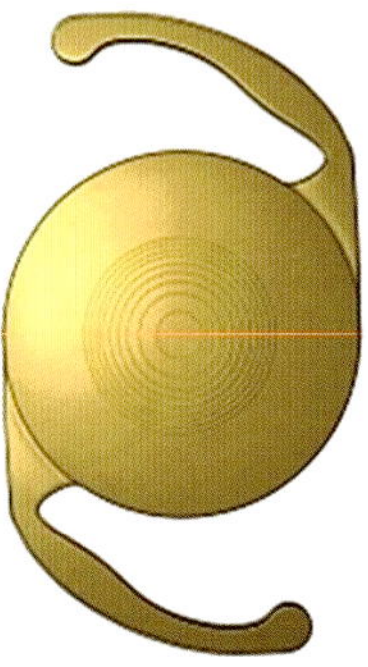

Fig. 7. ReSTOR apodized diffractive multifocal IOL (Alcon).

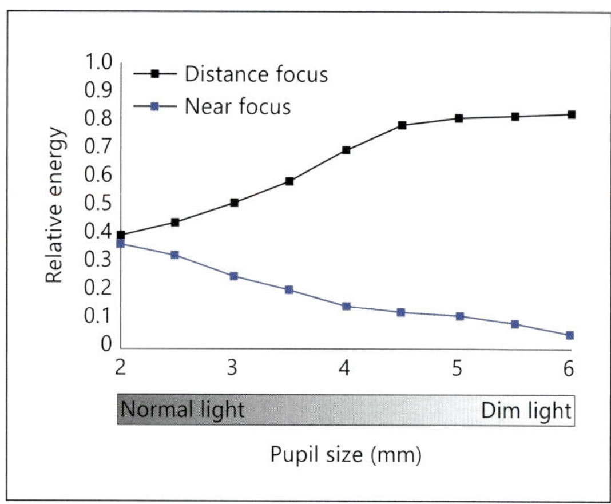

Fig. 8. Light distribution vs. pupil size with the Alcon ReSTOR lens.

cality should darken the part of the halo that is closer to the actual image border [12].

The need to reduce image confusion has been addressed with refractive designs as well. The recent multifocal model from Oculentis (Berlin, Germany) maintains only the inferior part of the near-refractive annulus, thus cutting the superior part of the confusion halo both in distant and in near vision [13] (fig. 10). Technically speaking, the near add might be positioned at any clock hour, as long as it is equally oriented in the two eyes.

All these approaches favour distant vision, and also have the purpose of reducing night glare and the starburst images around lights. Although neuroadaptation is required with multifocal IOLs, sometimes the perception of starbursts around lights frustrates patients with diffractive IOLs, and occasionally even causing IOL exchange to monofocal. With IOLs that have asymmetric light distribution, the low amount of light available for near vision is enough for reading high-contrast letters in normal lighting conditions, but low-contrast visual tasks in dim light may require to correct for near vision the brighter distant focus.

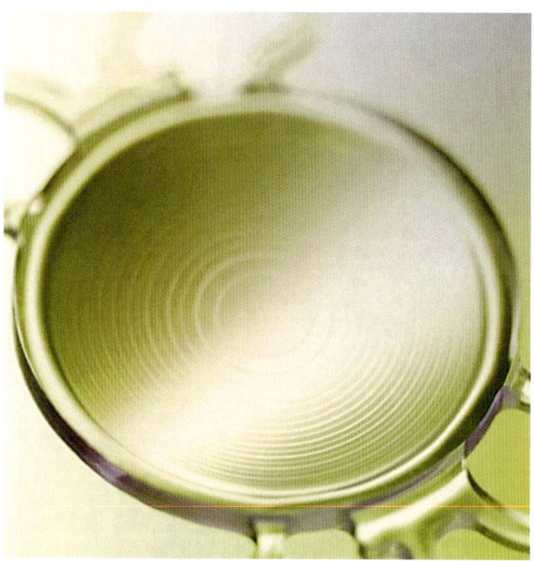

Fig. 9. FINE Vision trifocal IOL (PhysIOL).

Toric Multifocal Intraocular Lenses
To correct for preoperative corneal astigmatism, toric multifocal IOLs have become available from different manufacturers. Initial results in small clinical trials demonstrated their efficacy in providing the implanted eyes with good uncorrected vision both for distance and for near, similar as the spherical parent IOL [14, 15]. However, small rotation of the IOL can greatly decrease the correction of astigmatism, as happens with toric monofocal IOLs.

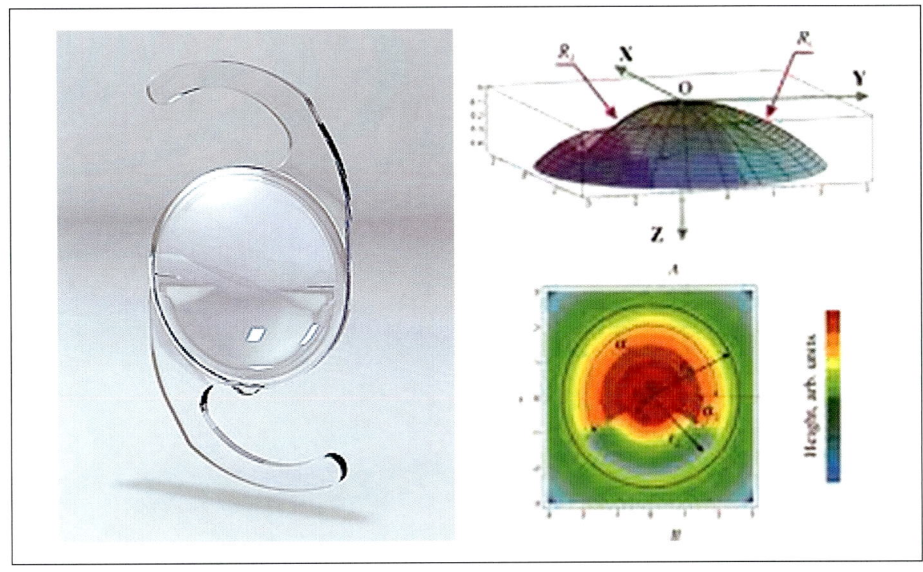

Fig. 10. Oculentis zonal refractive multifocal IOL.

Intermediate Vision with Multifocal Intraocular Lenses

Intermediate vision is a challenge with multifocal IOLs, and especially in computer reading [16]. IOLs with a +4-dpt add have an optimal reading distance of about 30 cm that might be too close, and visual acuity at 50–70 cm may be as low as 0.4 logMAR (fig. 11). However, the slight refraction disparity between the two eyes almost always encountered can help depth of field with bifocal IOLs. Bifocal IOLs with a +3-dpt add have become available after implementation of asphericity and of apodization, and are currently preferred to optimize vision at intermediate distances. The trifocal IOLs are a new and interesting approach to the problem of intermediate vision.

Multifocal Intraocular Lens Implant after Operation

With multifocal IOLs, success is good uncorrected vision both for distance and for near. Any problems reducing unaided vision will be perceived by the patient as surgery failure [17].

While spherical errors up to +0.5 dpt are well tolerated, myopic errors must be corrected while driving especially at night, and astigmatic errors must be corrected all day long. Since accuracy in IOL power calculation will only reduce the number of residual refractive errors, these and the possibility of laser corneal surgery should be communicated to the patient before cataract surgery. Patients who have already been operated for refractive corneal surgery are especially at risk of postoperative refractive error, and the feasibility of further corneal surgery must be checked before implanting a multifocal lens to give the patient proper advice.

Multifocal IOLs are very sensitive to posterior capsule opacification, and frequently require Nd:YAG posterior capsulotomy at an early stage as compared to monofocal IOLs [18]. This sensitivity probably comes from optical interference of the posterior capsule with the complex array of light rays emerging from multifocal IOLs, both diffractive and refractive. Laser posterior capsulotomy behind a multifocal IOL is by no means different than behind a monofocal IOL.

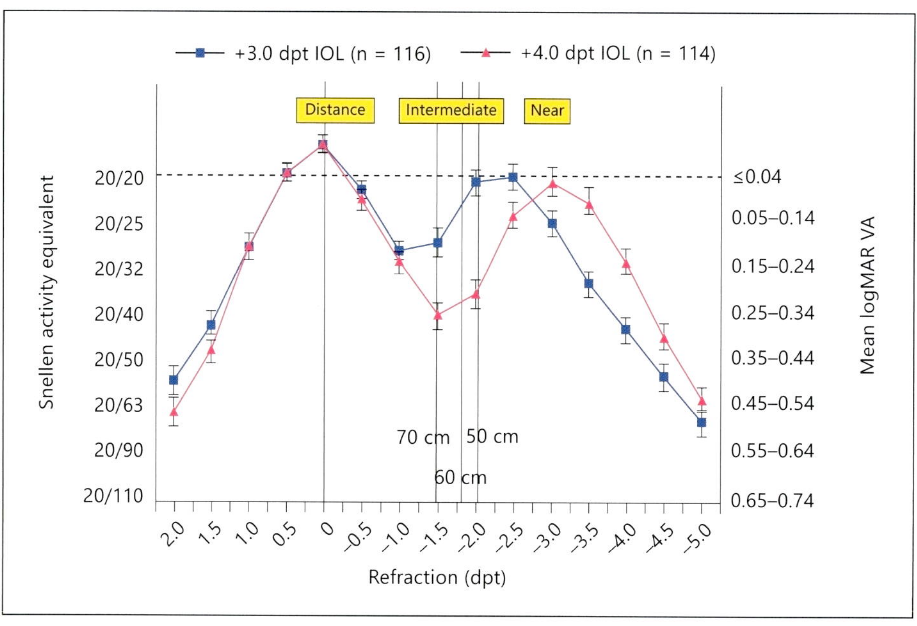

Fig. 11. Defocus curve indicating reduced intermediate vision with the +4-dpt add (www. sciencedirect.com).

For the multifocal IOL to work properly, the eye must have no other defects in image transmission or reception. Multifocal IOLs are not indicated in patients with corneal scarring or nubecolae, macular degeneration or problems of any kind. The problem arises with the possibility of macular degeneration occurring later in life that might reduce visual acuity particularly in eyes with multifocal IOLs. At the moment, multifocal IOLs cannot be recommended in eyes with soft drusen, as they may evolve in wet macular degeneration, or in eyes with concurrent macular atrophy of any kind.

Optical Quality with Multifocal Intraocular Lenses
Because of their double coaxial optics, multifocal IOLs provide lower optical quality as compared with monofocal IOLs [19]. Studies conducted with Hartmann-Shack aberrometers demonstrated complex pathways especially of spherical aberration that may be positive for smaller aperture diameters, and negative for larger, reducing point-spread function [20]. Double-pass machines also demonstrated reduction in point-spread function and MTF, and increase in the scattering index [21]. This reduction in MTF as compared with monofocal IOLs is the reason for the reduction in contrast sensitivity of implanted patients, which is the subjective counterpart of MTF. However, reduction in contrast sensitivity is rarely perceived by patients with normal retina, and is of importance only when contrast sensitivity is already reduced by other comorbidities, i.e. high myopia [22].

Visual Results and Patient Satisfaction
By analyzing the published literature, the Cochrane review prepared by Calladine et al. [23] found only 16 papers reporting well-organized and conducted studies, with 1,608 participants. The emerging evidence is that multifocal IOLs

Table 1. Preferred reading distance for a few popular multifocal IOLs

Model	Far/near	Add at lens plane, dpt	Add at spectacle plane, dpt	Reading distance, cm
ReSTOR +4	apodized	+4	+3.2	30
Tecnis MF	50:50	+4	+3.0	30
Acri.LISA	66:33	+3.75	+3.0	32
ReSTOR +3	apodized	+3	+2.4	35
SeeLens MF	apodized	+3	+2.4	35

provide the same uncorrected and corrected distance vision as monofocal IOLs, but definitely better near vision. Contrast sensitivity was similar with either IOL type when analyzed with the Pelli-Robson chart, but it was better with monofocal IOLs when analyzed with the FACT chart. The risk for reporting some glare and halos was almost double with multifocals, although rarely disturbing. Patient satisfaction was difficult to assess and compare because of the different methods of investigation adopted by the different studies, and because patient expectations may affect the reported satisfaction level, but it was slightly better with multifocals.

Another survey published in 2011 found that diffractive multifocal IOLs provided the same distant vision as refractive multifocal IOLs, but better near vision [24]. The preferred reading distance depended on the near add, and is reported in table 1 for a few popular multifocal IOLs.

Spectacle independency was not universally obtained across the examined studies, both because of residual refractive error (toric multifocal lenses were not available), poor intermediate vision, and because of personal needs and opinions of patients. However, spectacle independency of patients with multifocal IOLs was 1.7 times that of patients with monofocal IOL. The same meta-analysis found the perception of halos with multifocal IOLs to be higher than with monofocal IOLs, but that of diffractive multifocal IOL is the lowest (table 2).

Table 2. Patient satisfaction and halo as compared to monofocal lens [24]

Lens type	Patient satisfaction		Perception of haloes	
	odds ratio	95% CI	odds ratio	95% CI
Monofocal	1	reference	1	reference
Multifocal	1.03	0.9–1.17	1.13	0.91–1.39
Diffractive MF	1.05	0.85–1.31	0.71	0.48–1.05

Pseudoaccommodative Intraocular Lenses

Pseudoaccommodation means the IOL power of a monofocal lens has the ability to change from distance vision to near vision. The quest for restoring accommodation by special IOL design is long-standing. The first studies of Cumming date back to 1990, culminating in the first pseudoaccommodative IOL FDA approved in 2003, the Crystalens AT 45 [25]. At the moment, there are three pseudoaccommodative IOLs of interest: two are based on a single optics approach, the third on a dual optics approach.

Single-Optic Pseudoaccommodative Intraocular Lenses

The principle underlying this approach is the forward movement of IOL optics during near vision, a movement occasionally demonstrated with IOLs. To facilitate this movement, a special haptic design is required. The Crystalens HD

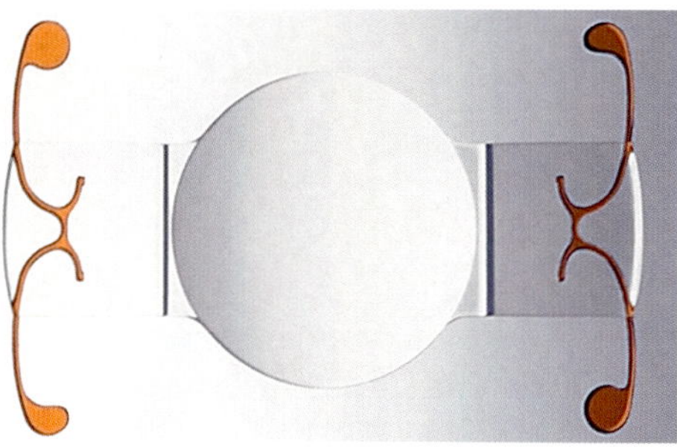

Fig. 12. The Crystalens HD pseudoaccommodative IOL (Bausch & Lomb).

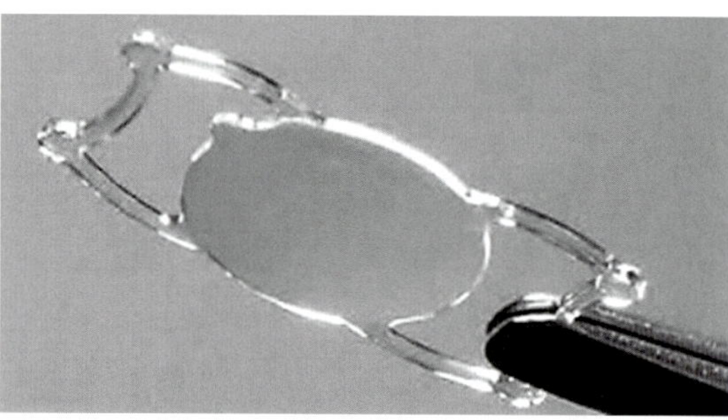

Fig. 13. The Tetraflex pseudoaccommodative IOL (Lenstec).

IOL (Bausch & Lomb, Rochester, N.Y., USA) is the latest version of Cumming's model (fig. 12): it is made of silicone, with polyamide haptics enlargement, and has two hinges near the optic-haptic junction to favour the forward movement of the IOL during near vision [25]. The Tetraflex IOL (Lenstec, St. Petersburg, Fla., USA) is a hydrophilic acrylic IOL with weak haptics to favor optics movement that provided interesting results in clinical investigations [26] (fig. 13).

During near vision, the contraction of the ciliary body will reduce the diameter of the capsular bag, compressing IOL haptics. Haptics compression and the posterior vitreous pressure will induce a forward movement of the IOL optics because of the special haptics design. The more anterior position of the optics will increase the effective dioptric power according to the amount of forward shift and to the base dioptric power of the IOL. For this process to be effective, a forward shift of almost 1 mm is required for an IOL of at least +18-dpt power.

The Crystalens series has been studied extensively, and it has been found to provide up to 1.5 dpt of pseudoaccommodation in clinical practice [27–29], although this is not much different from the 0.75–1.0 dpt that can be observed with microincision IOLs. In addition, the forward movement of the IOL is controversial: some authors demonstrated it to happen even after laser posterior capsulotomy [30], others were not able to demonstrate any

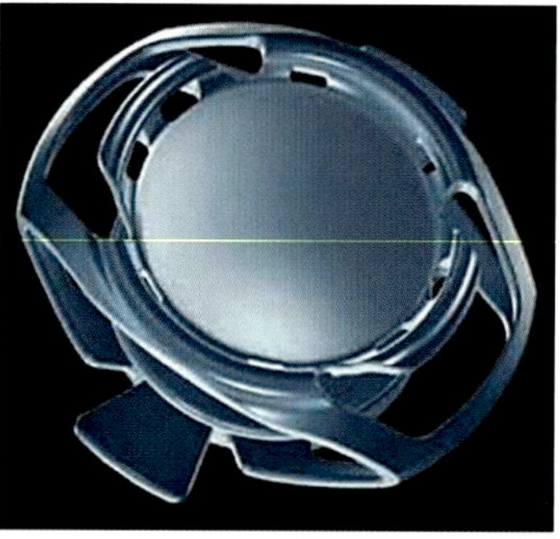

Fig. 14. The Synchrony pseudoaccommodative dual-optic IOL (AMO).

movement by careful ultrasound studies [31]. At the moment, this IOL is considered to offer good distance and intermediate vision, but spectacles are usually required for close reading.

Dual-Optic Pseudoaccommodative Intraocular Lens

The Synchrony IOL (Abbott, Santa Ana, Calif., USA) is a monofocal IOL based on the dual optics principle (fig. 14). It is composed of silicone and has a +32-dpt anterior optic that is 5.5 mm wide, along with a 6-mm posterior optic that varies in power based on the patient's needs and is usually negative. The two optics are connected by spring haptics, and the whole device is 9.5 × 9.8 mm in size and designed to fill the capsular bag [32, 33]. During near reading, the anterior

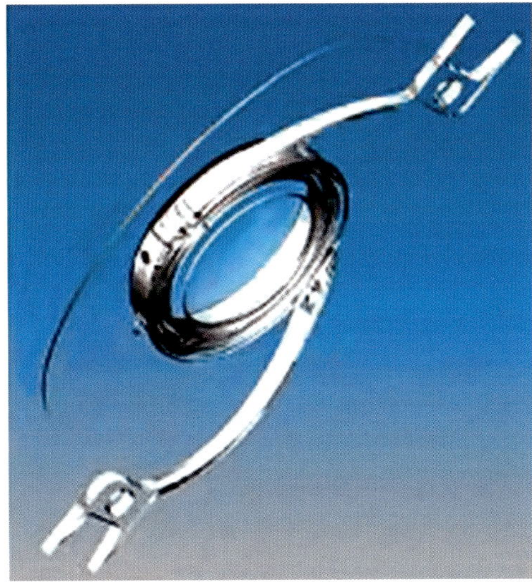

Fig. 15. The Nu-Lens accommodative IOL.

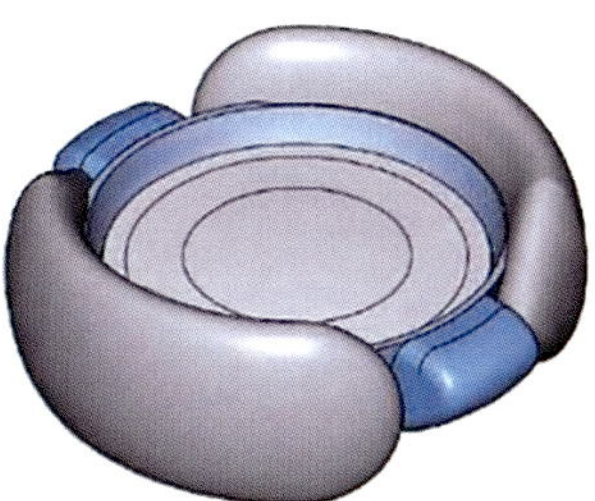

Fig. 16. The FluidVision lens (PowerVision).

optics is supposed to move forward, obtaining as much as 2.2 dpt of pseudoaccommodation. However, reported results still indicate the need for small near add for close reading.

Future Intraocular Lenses

Many new IOLs are entering preclinical or clinical studies, and many are in the pipeline. Out of these, we selected the concepts that may be of interest for the future.

A fluid IOL optics might change its shape according to selected stimuli, and provide pseudo-accommodation. The fluid content is usually liq-

uid silicone, hosted in a thin silicone bag of different shapes when relaxed and compressed by ciliary muscle action. The Dyna-Curve (Nu-Lens, Ltd., Herzliya Pituah, Israel) is probably the best known example of this approach (fig. 15), and provided good results in the initial clinical trials [34]. The FluidVision lens (PowerVision, Inc., Belmont, Calif., USA) is another approach still awaiting clinical trials (fig. 16).

Another approach is lens refilling. With this technique, the capsular bag is evacuated through a small capsular opening to be then refilled with an elastic polymer that responds to an adequate change in surface curvature according to the varying zonular tension [35]. Ideally, the material should be cytotoxic upon direct contact in order to prevent after-cataract, but should not release toxic substances into the surroundings and should not leak into the anterior chamber before polymerization.

Various alternative approaches have been presented for capsular bag refilling: from an inflatable silicone balloon filled with a liquid silicone polymer [36] to silicone plugs for sealing the mini-capsulorhexis required for cataract removal and liquid silicone injection [37]. With both the balloon and plug approaches, however, the accommodative amplitude achieved in study animals was only a fraction of the expected values, decreasing over time, and secondary cataract developed in all eyes. In addition, toxicity problems have never been addressed in full. The recent introduction of femtosecond laser technology in cataract surgery, providing capsular openings of any size and location, might prompt new studies about lens refilling.

Auto-focusing IOLs are IOLs powered by their own power cell and computer chip embedded inside [38]. They are rechargeable and fully programmable, allowing to adapt its optical power as the patient's visual needs change. The Elenza IOL (Roanoke, Va., USA) combines nanotechnology, artificial intelligence (neural network-based memory), and advanced electronics to seamlessly autofocus an optic from far to near without movement by changing the molecular configuration of the liquid crystal the IOL optic is made of. The IOL relies on individual pupillary response to far and near vision to automatically trigger accommodation. This technology is fascinating and promising, and investigators are trying to solve the residual problems.

Disclosure Statement

The author is a consultant for Bausch & Lomb, and has received research grants from Hanita Lenses, Acritec-Zeiss, and SIFI.

References

1 Bellucci R, Giardini P: Pseudoaccommodation with the 3M diffractive multifocal intraocular lens: a refraction study of 52 subjects. J Cataract Refract Surg 1993;19:32–35.
2 Ravalico G, Baccara F, Bellavitis A: Refractive bifocal intraocular lens and pupillary diameter. J Cataract Refract Surg 1992;18:594–597.
3 Bellucci R: Multifocal intraocular lenses. Curr Opin Ophthalmol 2005;16: 33–37.
4 Kawamorita T, Uozato H: Modulation transfer function and pupil size in multifocal and monofocal intraocular lenses in vitro. J Cataract Refract Surg 2005;31: 2379–2385.
5 Portney V: Light distribution in diffractive multifocal optics and its optimization. J Cataract Refract Surg 2011;37: 2053–2059.
6 Muñoz G, Albarrán-Diego C, Cerviño A, Ferrer-Blasco T, García-Lázaro S: Visual and optical performance with the ReZoom multifocal intraocular lens. Eur J Ophthalmol 2012;22:356–362.
7 Mester U, Hunold W, Wesendahl T, Kaymak H: Functional outcomes after implantation of Tecnis ZM900 and Array SA40 multifocal intraocular lenses. J Cataract Refract Surg 2007;33:1033–1040.
8 Alfonso JF, Fernández-Vega L, Ortí S, Montés-Micó R: Refractive lens exchange with the Acri.Twin asymmetric diffractive bifocal intraocular lens system. Eur J Ophthalmol 2010;20:509–516.
9 Kohnen T, Allen D, Boureau C, Dublineau P, Hartmann C, Mehdorn E, Rozot P, Tassinari G: European multicenter study of the AcrySof ReSTOR apodized diffractive intraocular lens. Ophthalmology 2006;113:584.e1.

10 Vega F, Alba-Bueno F, Millán MS: Energy distribution between distance and near images in apodized diffractive multifocal intraocular lenses. Invest Ophthalmol Vis Sci 2011;52:5695–5701.
11 Choi J, Schwiegerling J: Optical performance measurement and night driving simulation of ReSTOR, ReZoom, and Tecnis multifocal intraocular lenses in a model eye. J Refract Surg 2008;24:218–222.
12 Gatinel D, Pagnoulle C, Houbrechts Y, Gobin L: Design and qualification of a diffractive trifocal optical profile for intraocular lenses. J Cataract Refract Surg 2011;37:2060–2067.
13 Muñoz G, Albarrán-Diego C, Ferrer-Blasco T, Sakla HF, García-Lázaro S: Visual function after bilateral implantation of a new zonal refractive aspheric multifocal intraocular lens. J Cataract Refract Surg 2011;37:2043–2052.
14 Mojzis P, Piñero DP, Studeny P, Tomás J, Korda V, Plaza AB, Alió JL: Comparative analysis of clinical outcomes obtained with a new diffractive multifocal toric intraocular lens implanted through two types of corneal incision. J Refract Surg 2011;27:648–657.
15 Visser N, Nuijts RM, de Vries NE, Bauer NJ: Visual outcomes and patient satisfaction after cataract surgery with toric multifocal intraocular lens implantation. J Cataract Refract Surg 2011;37:2034–2042.
16 Rabsilber TM, Rudalevicius P, Jasinskas V, Holzer MP, Auffarth GU: Influence of +3.00 and +4.00 D near addition on functional outcomes of a refractive multifocal intraocular lens model. J Cataract Refract Surg 2013;39: 350–357.

17 Leccisotti A: Secondary procedures after presbyopic lens exchange. J Cataract Refract Surg 2004;30:1461–1465.
18 Shah VC, Russo C, Cannon R, Davidson R, Taravella MJ: Incidence of Nd:YAG capsulotomy after implantation of AcrySof multifocal and monofocal intraocular lenses: a case controlled study. J Refract Surg 2010;26: 565–568.
19 Santhiago MR, Wilson SE, Netto MV, Ghanen RC, Monteiro ML, Bechara SJ, Espana EM, Mello GR, Kara N Jr: Modulation transfer function and optical quality after bilateral implantation of a +3.00 versus a +4.00 D multifocal intraocular lens. J Cataract Refract Surg 2012;38:215–220.
20 Santhiago MR, Netto MV, Barreto J, Gomes BA, Schaefer A, Kara-Junior N: Wavefront analysis and modulation transfer function of three multifocal intraocular lenses. Indian J Ophthalmol 2010;58:109–113.
21 Moreno LJ, Piñero DP, Alió JL, Fimia A, Plaza AB: Double-pass system analysis of the visual outcomes and optical performance of an apodized diffractive multifocal intraocular lens. J Cataract Refract Surg 2010;36:2048–2055.
22 Alfonso JF, Fernández-Vega L, Ortí S, Ferrer-Blasco T, Montés-Micò R: Differences in visual performance of AcrySof ReSTOR IOL in high and low myopic eyes. Eur J Ophthalmol 2010;20:333–339.
23 Calladine D, Evans JR, Shah S, Leyland M: Multifocal versus monofocal intraocular lenses after cataract extraction. Cochrane Database Syst Rev 2012; 9:CD003169.
24 Cochener B, Lafuma A, Khoshnood B, Courouve L, Berdeaux G: Comparison of outcomes with multifocal intraocular lenses: a meta-analysis. Clin Ophthalmol 2011;5:45–56.

25 Dick HB: Accommodative intraocular lenses: current status. Curr Opin Ophthalmol 2005;16:8–26.

26 Sanders DR, Sanders ML, Tetraflex Presbyopic IOL Study Group: US FDA clinical trial of the Tetraflex potentially accommodating IOL: comparison to concurrent age-matched monofocal controls. J Refract Surg 2010;26:723–730.

27 Tahir HJ, Tong JL, Geissler S, Vedamurthy I, Schor CM: Effects of accommodation training on accommodation and depth of focus in an eye implanted with a crystalens intraocular lens. J Refract Surg 2010;26:772–779.

28 Alió JL, Piñero DP, Plaza-Puche AB: Visual outcomes and optical performance with a monofocal intraocular lens and a new-generation single-optic accommodating intraocular lens. J Cataract Refract Surg 2010;36:1656–1664.

29 Hantera MM, Hamed AM, Fekry Y, Shoheib EA: Initial experience with an accommodating intraocular lens: controlled prospective study. J Cataract Refract Surg 2010;36:1167–1172.

30 Alió JL, Tavolato M, De la Hoz F, Claramonte P, Rodríguez-Prats JL, Galal A: Near vision restoration with refractive lens exchange and pseudoaccommodating and multifocal refractive and diffractive intraocular lenses: comparative clinical study. J Cataract Refract Surg 2004;30:2494–2503.

31 Koeppl C, Findl O, Menapace R, Kriechbaum K, Wirtitsch M, Buehl W, Sacu S, Drexler W: Pilocarpine-induced shift of an accommodating intraocular lens: AT-45 Crystalens. J Cataract Refract Surg 2005;31:1290–1297.

32 McLeod SD, Vargas LG, Portney V, Ting A: Synchrony dual-optic accommodating intraocular lens. 1. Optical and biomechanical principles and design considerations. J Cataract Refract Surg 2007;33:37–46.

33 Alió JL, Plaza-Puche AB, Montalban R, Ortega P: Near visual outcomes with single-optic and dual-optic accommodating intraocular lenses. J Cataract Refract Surg 2012;38:1568–1575.

34 Ben-Nun J: The NuLens accommodating intraocular lens. Ophthalmol Clin North Am 2006;19:129–134.

35 Koopmans SA, Terwee T, van Kooten TG: Prevention of capsular opacification after accommodative lens refilling surgery in rabbits. Biomaterials 2011;32:5743–5755.

36 Nishi O, Hara T, Hara T, Sakka Y, Hayashi F, Nakamae K, Yamada Y: Refilling the lens with an inflatable endocapsular balloon: surgical procedure in animal eyes. Graefes Arch Clin Exp Ophthalmol 1992;230:47–55.

37 Nishi O, Nishi K: Accommodation amplitude after lens refilling with injectable silicone by sealing the capsule with a plug in primates. Arch Ophthalmol 1998;116:1358–1361.

38 Haiden AF: Electronic IOLs: the future of cataract surgery. Eye World, Feb 2012.

Roberto Bellucci, MD
Ophthalmic Unit, Department of Neurosciences
Hospital and University of Verona, Borgo Trento Hospital
IT–37126 Verona (Italy)
E-Mail roberto.bellucci@ospedaleuniverona.it

Güell JL (ed): Cataract. ESASO Course Series. Basel, Karger, 2013, vol 3, pp 38–55
DOI: 10.1159/000350902

An Introduction to Intraocular Lenses: Material, Optics, Haptics, Design and Aberration

Roberto Bellucci

Ophthalmic Unit, Department of Neurosciences, Hospital and University of Verona, Verona, Italy

Abstract

Several intraocular lens (IOL) materials and types are currently available. Polymethyl methacrylate IOLs used to be the gold standard, but the inability of folding limits their use to selected countries and patients. Silicone IOLs were used more in the past because they are less suitable for microincisions. Foldable hydrophobic acrylic is the most popular material, which is also available in yellow (blue light absorbing) models and several IOL shapes. Although a very effective and safe material, water penetration producing glistenings and some dysphotopsia has been reported with some IOL types. Foldable hydrophilic material is widely employed in Europe, and especially for microincision cataract surgery lenses because of its plasticity, even if rare optics opacification and higher posterior capsular opacification rates have been reported in the past. Single-piece IOLs are the most employed in modern cataract surgery, but 3-piece IOLs are preferred for sulcus implantation and in infants. The aspheric design to correct or to control spherical aberration in implanted eyes is now the rule after the problems of centration we had before the capsulorhexis era were solved. However, the optical quality of pseudophakic eyes will depend not only on aberration control, but also on good media transparency and low light scattering.

Definition and History

An intraocular lens (IOL) is a lens implanted in the eye to treat large refractive errors. IOLs usually consist of small optics with side structures, called haptics, to hold the lens in place within the capsular bag inside the eye. The most common type of IOL is inserted into the capsular bag after cataract (lens) removal and is known as 'aphakic IOL'. The second type of IOL, more commonly known as a phakic IOL, is placed inside the eye without removing the existing natural lens, to correct large refractive errors.

The first IOL was implanted by Sir Harold Ridley on 29 November 1949, at St Thomas' Hospital in London (fig. 1). That first IOL was manufactured from polymethyl methacrylate (PMMA, also known as Perspex or Plexiglas), that was chosen because Ridley noticed it was inert in the eyes of RAF pilots [1]. The IOL concept spread slowly until the 1970s, when new and lighter posterior chamber lenses were designed, introducing polypropylene haptics for ciliary sulcus fixation [2]. Currently, there are several types and models of IOLs designed for specific purposes.

Destination	Capsular bag, ciliary sulcus, scleral fixation, iris fixation, angle supported
Overall design	3 piece/1 piece
Overall length	10–13 mm
Optics material	Rigid (PMMA), flexible (silicone), foldable (hydrophobic acrylic, hydrophilic acrylic), Collamer
Refraction index	1.42–1.55
Optics shape	Biconvex, plano-convex, meniscus
Optics diameter	5–7 mm
Optics design	Spherical, aspheric, toric multifocal, multifocal toric
Optics color	Transparent, tinted
Haptics properties	3 piece/1 piece (PMMA, PVDF, polyamide, 2, 3, 4, 6 haptics)
Type of implantation	Injectable, not injectable
Type of packaging	Pre-loaded, not pre-loaded

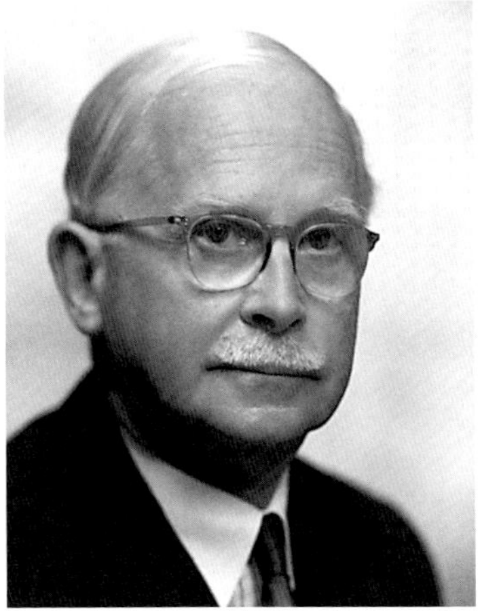

Fig. 1. Sir Harold Ridley.

An Overview of Current Models

The several types of IOLs currently available can be differentiated in several ways, the most important of which are shown in table 1.

The ideal IOL should offer advantages both to the surgeon and to the patient. The surgeon looks for easiness of implantation and lack of intraoperative complications, the patient asks for good and long-lasting vision, and for refractive stabili-ty. In recent years, a tendency has developed preferring foldable IOLs and especially those suitable for microincision cataract surgery (MICS), i.e. those IOLs that can be implanted through sub-2 mm incision. These lenses are usually hydrophilic acrylic single-piece IOLs. IOL materials are defined hydrophobic or hydrophilic according to the angle a drop of water makes with respect to the material surface. The more acute this angle is, the more hydrophilic the material is defined. Although hydrophilic lenses must be packaged immersed in normal saline, there is nothing against packaging the lenses made of hydrophobic materials wet. Every IOL is immersed in water once inside the eye.

Materials

Polymethyl Methacrylate
PMMA was the first material used for IOLs (fig. 2). It is a rigid, non-foldable, hydrophobic (water content <1%) material. The refractive index is 1.49, and the usual optic diameter is 5–7 mm. PMMA IOLs are usually single piece, with fragile and low memory haptics, unless a compression molding production is employed. PMMA lenses are usually thin as the rigidity of the material bal-

ances the low refraction index. Because of the required large incision, PMMA IOLs are seldom preferred today. They are currently used in developing countries because of the low cost, and in children given the proven long life in implanted eyes [3].

As any material immersed in water, PMMA may be penetrated by aqueous humor sometimes. This will cause small vacuoles to appear within the lens optic, a phenomenon called 'glistenings'. Glistenings are very rare with PMMA IOLs, but they have been observed, and at least on one occasion have caused optic opacification [4].

Silicone

Polymers of silicone and oxygen have been employed as IOL material since 1984 [5], with the purpose of implanting the IOL through an incision narrower than IOL diameter (fig. 3). Silicone is hydrophobic, with a contact angle with water of 99°, higher than that of hydrophobic acrylic material. Silicone IOLs must be handled dry if folder and holder forceps are employed for implantation, because it is slippery when wet. Giant cell coverage of this material is similar to that of hydrophobic acrylic IOLs. The refractive index is usually between 1.41 and 1.46, the optic diameter is 5.5–6.5 mm. Current models are 3 piece, with PMMA, polyvinyl difluoride (PVDF) or polyamide haptics. Because of the low refractive index, the optics is rather thick, requiring incisions larger than 3.2 mm to implant higher-power lenses. Recently, injectors for 3-piece silicone lenses have been developed, allowing better and safer handling. However, the abrupt opening of silicone IOLs inside the anterior chamber remains a problem for surgeons. Silicone lenses have been suspected to favor bacterial adhesion, with increased risk for postoperative infection – an item never demonstrated in surgical setting [6]. After implantation, the anterior capsule rim opacifies quickly (fig. 4), while the posterior capsule may remain clear for many years. Despite the low posterior capsular opacification (PCO)

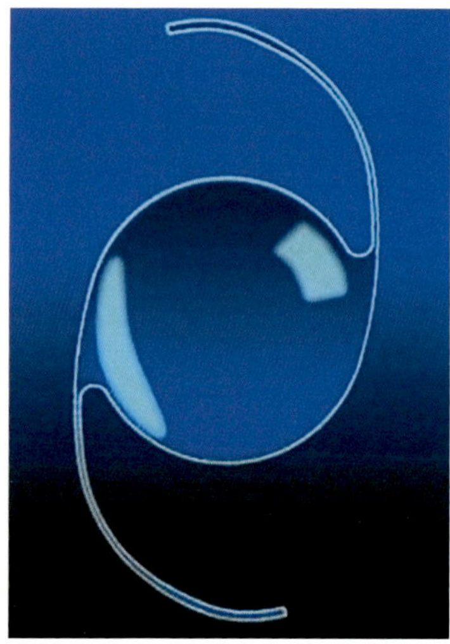

Fig. 2. PMMA IOL of recent design.

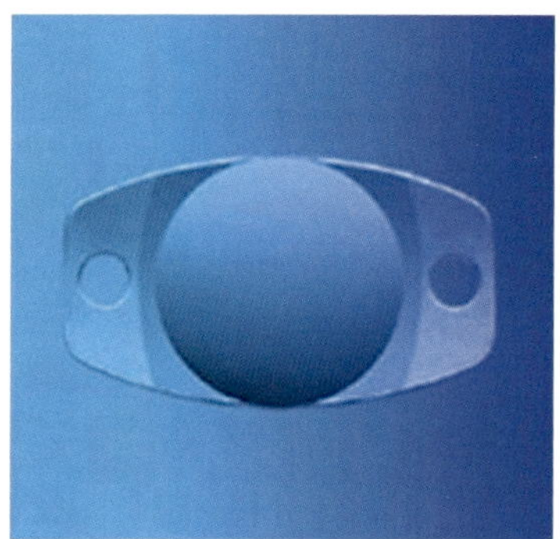

Fig. 3. Silicone plate-haptic IOL that was introduced in 1984.

rate and the good resistance to Nd:YAG laser shots, silicone is less used today because it is not suitable for MICS. Recently, a two-component silicone IOL was designed, in which power can be adjusted after implantation through UV exposure. The light-adjustable lens is entering clinical practice, and the ability to correct for spherical and cylindrical errors might overcome the 3.2 mm incision disadvantages [7, 8].

We should remember that the lens capsule will never adhere to silicone, and therefore the optics will be kept in place by the haptics and by capsule coalescence. Therefore, we should refrain from implanting silicone lenses with damaged haptics, an issue unfortunately emerging only after the lens optics is inside the eye. When removing the lens, cutting the haptics will impede any extraction through small incision.

Silicone can be penetrated by aqueous humor too, and glistenings may appear within silicone optics [9]. However, the main problem with silicone IOLs is the adherence of silicone droplets in the case of silicone oil tamponade after retinal detachment repair [10]. These eyes always require Nd:YAG posterior capsulotomy, and silicone droplets deposit onto the posterior IOL surface after silicone oil removal, causing IOL explantation and exchange. For this reason, silicone material may not be preferred in highly myopic eyes that are at increased risk for posterior segment surgery.

Hydrophobic Foldable Acrylic
Hydrophobic foldable acrylic materials are a series of copolymers of acrylate and methacrylate derived from rigid PMMA, with the purpose of making them foldable and durable. The typical angle of contact with water is 73° [11]. Hydrophobic foldable acrylic lenses can be folded, pushed, and pulled, always regaining their original shape in a matter of seconds [12].

Hydrophobic acrylic foldable lenses were introduced in 1993 with the first Acrysof 3-piece lens (Alcon, Forth Worth, Tex., USA; fig. 5), and have been probably the most successful IOLs thereafter. Hydrophobic acrylic IOLs are available in 3-piece or 1-piece designs (fig. 6), optic diameter between 5.5 and 7.0 mm, overall length between 12 and 13 mm, transparent or yellow, with a refractive index between 1.44 and 1.55. Hydrophobic acrylic foldable lenses are easy to implant, however require at least a 2.2-mm incision. Some of them can receive permanent fingerprints or scratches by implantation instruments, while others claim to be harder. As a common feature,

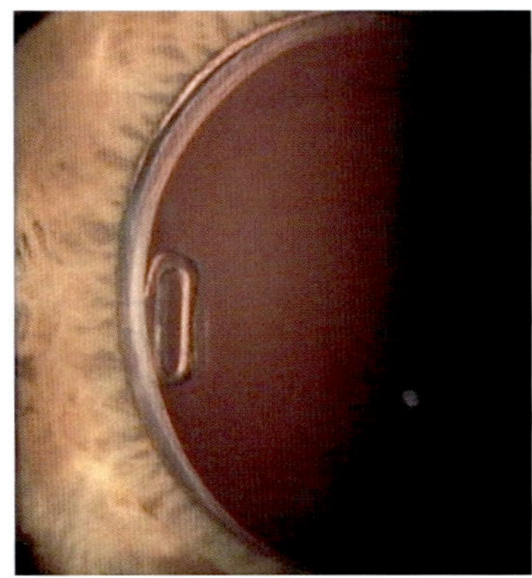

Fig. 4. Fibrosis of the anterior capsule rim with silicone IOL.

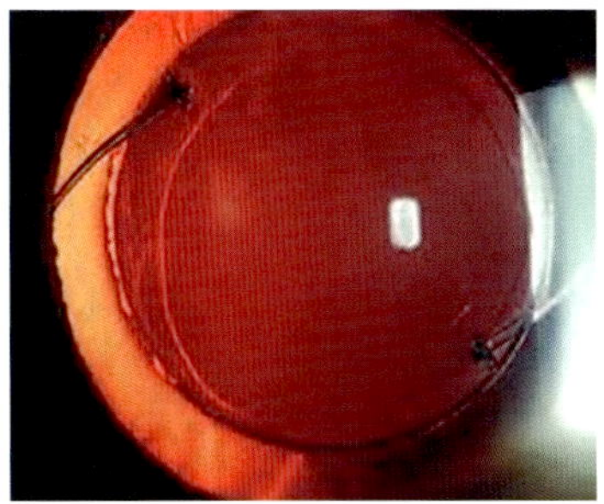

Fig. 5. Three-piece foldable hydrophobic acrylic IOL.

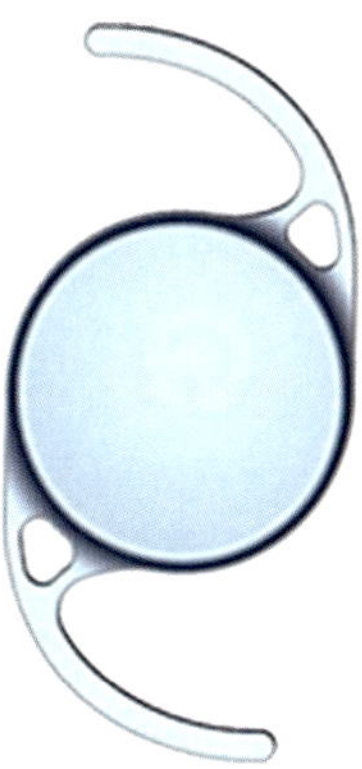

Fig. 6. One-piece foldable hydrophobic acrylic IOL.

these lenses show low tendency to self-centering, and care must be taken to position them properly at implantation.

In the postoperative period, they elicit low degrees of posterior capsule opacification and receive little damage from Nd:YAG laser posterior capsulotomy. Moreover, they show little tendency to attract silicone droplets after silicone oil tamponade, albeit hydrophilic acrylic material is still better. At the moment (2012) hydrophilic acrylic IOLs are the most popular worldwide, especially in the US because of the FDA approval.

Hydrophobic foldable intraocular lenses have been associated with photopsias more frequently than other types of acrylic IOLs, an item related to low anterior curvatures and high refractive index [13, 14]. In addition, some of them are easily penetrated by aqueous humor, and develop glistenings in the form of water microvacuoles within the IOL optics (fig. 7), a problem not pertaining to all hydrophobic foldable materials [15]. Glistenings seem to be clinically important only when dense or with special (multifocal) design. To overcome this drawback, new materials have been introduced that are prehydrated to equilibrium and will not accept further water, thus avoiding the formation of glistenings. These IOLs are hydrophobic because the contact angle with water is that of hydrophobic acrylic, but are packaged in BSS to absorb the eventual 4% water content before implantation [16].

Hydrophilic Foldable Acrylic
Hydrophilic acrylic materials are composed of a mixture of hydroxyethylmethacrylate (poly-HEMA) and hydrophilic acrylic monomer [17]. Compounds specifically prepared for IOLs appeared at the end of the 1980s and underwent several modifications thereafter, giving rise to a list of materials of different copolymers and water content, usually between 18 and 26%. A typical refractive index is 1.43, and some materials

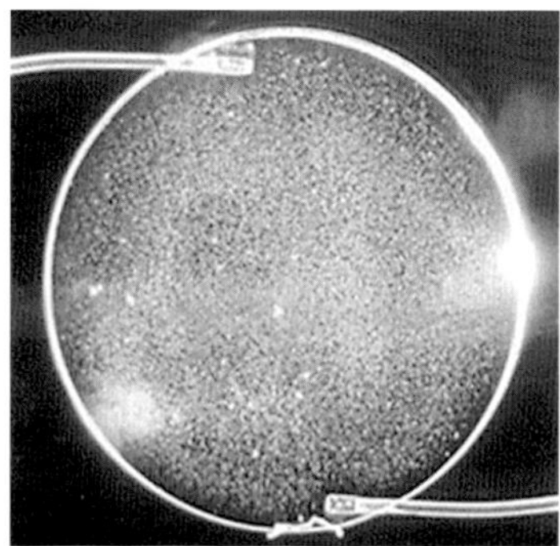

Fig. 7. Optic microvacuoles known as glistenings.

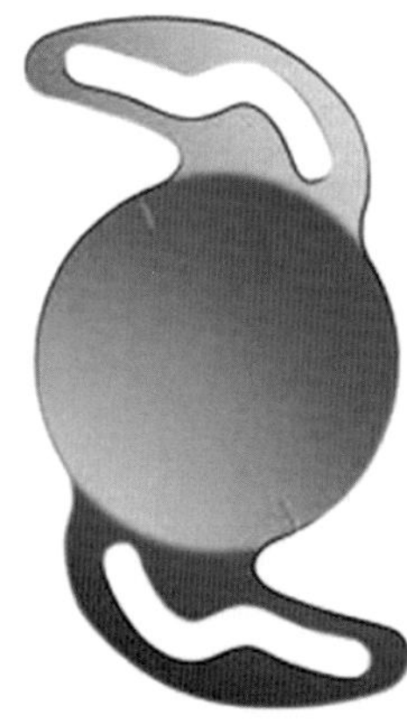

Fig. 8. Foldable hydrophilic acrylic IOL.

can be yellow tinted (fig. 8). Hydrophilic acrylic lenses are soft, somewhat compressible, and have excellent biocompatibility because of their hydrophilic surface. The contact angle with water is lower than 50°. Most IOLs are single piece, and designed for capsular bag implantation with few exceptions. Hydrophilic acrylic material is the easiest to handle, with low tendency to receive scratches from instruments or damage from Nd:YAG laser shots. They can be implanted through sub-2-mm incisions and are the ideal lenses for MICS [18] (fig. 9). The number and shape of haptics varies widely, but these lenses are rarely found displaced if properly implanted. In the postoperative period, the induction of photopsias is low, but the PCO rate is considered to be higher than with other materials, although recent research seems to contradict this statement [19]. Hydrophilic acrylic material is considered weaker than hydrophobic, with lower resistance to capsular bag contraction [20]. Therefore, they may not be preferred when high contraction forces are anticipated, as in some eyes with pseudoexfoliation.

The main concern with hydrophilic acrylic lenses is optic opacification due to calcium deposits, a rare event that led to IOL exchange in a number of patients (fig. 10). In the past, this calcification has been associated with certain IOL types and/or certain viscoelastic substances, but its mechanism is still unclear [21, 22]. Hydrophilic IOLs are very popular in Europe because of the easy handling, the sub-2-mm implantation, the low risk for capsular bag damage during implantation, and the improving results with PCO.

Collamer

Collamer is the name of the material used exclusively in making STAAR® Company phakic and aphakic lenses, including the Visian ICL (fig. 11). The name comes from the combination of 'collagen' and 'polymer'. IOLs made of Collamer are highly biocompatible, and easy to implant because of the softness of the material and the gentle unfolding [23]. Water content is very high, at about 40%, which makes this material very soft and also suitable for aphakic IOLs.

The collagen in the Collamer attracts fibronectin, a substance found naturally in the eye. A layer of fibronectin forms around the lens, inhibiting white cell adhesion to the lens. This coating prevents the lens from being identified as a foreign object, and the lens remains unnoticed and 'quiet in the eye' indefinitely. In addition, like the collagen it contains, Collamer carries a slight nega-

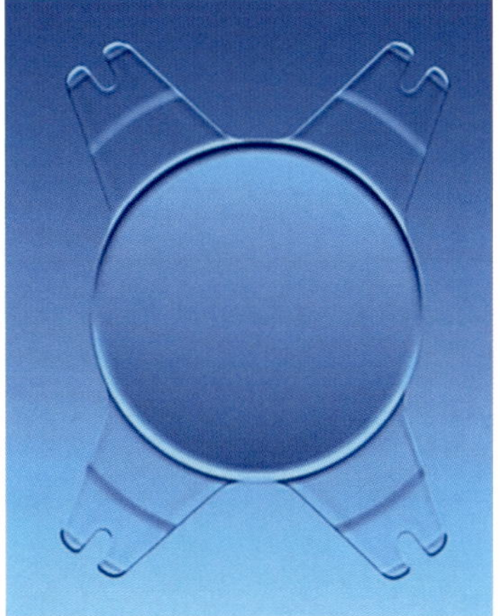

Fig. 9. Foldable hydrophilic acrylic microincision IOL.

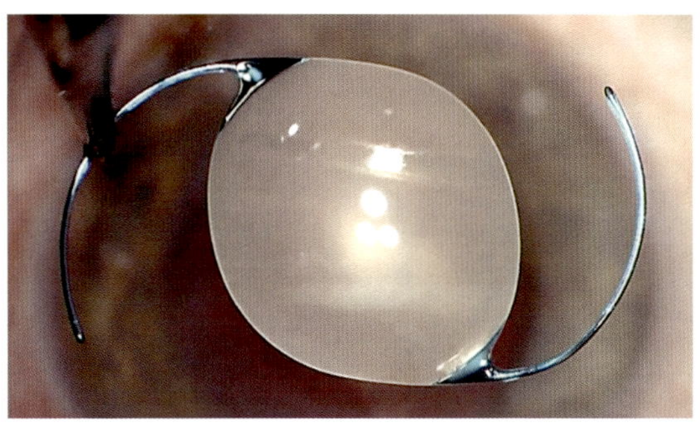

Fig. 10. IOL opacification due to calcium deposits.

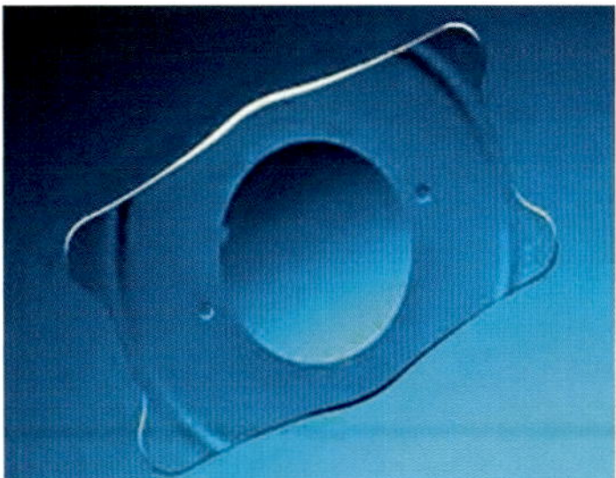

Fig. 11. Collamer IOL.

tive ionic charge that pushes away the negatively charged proteins from the lens, keeping it clean and clear [24].

Selected Properties of Intraocular Lens Materials
The different materials show differences that might influence IOL selection, according to surgeon's preferences, the most important of which are listed below.

Light reflection is more pronounced with some hydrophobic materials, because of the different physical properties of the two media – aqueous humor and IOL surface. The same hydrophobic foldable acrylic material has been associated with internal light reflections possibly causing dysphotopsia [25].

Dysphotopsia is the name of all the visible phenomena experienced by pseudophakic patients. Positive dysphotopsia usually appears as an arc of light mimicking the IOL border, even though covered by an anterior capsule rim. Negative dysphotopsia is the appearance of a dark crescent or halo. Dysphotopsia can happen with any IOL material, although hydrophilic acrylic is considered of advantage [26].

Visible light absorption varies across materials. Silicone and hydrophilic acrylic materials are considered less transparent than hydrophobic acrylic, but still much more transparent than a transparent human lens. In addition, some IOLs include a yellow pigment to reduce or block blue or violet visible radiation that may be harmful for the retina. Materials absorbing visible light are very controversial to date; however, they reduce the postoperative glare often reported by pseudophakic patients [27].

Ultraviolet light absorption is a feature of every IOL, as all of them contain a chromophore designed to absorb UV radiation below 400 nm [28].

Color rendering of IOL materials is defined by the Abbe number. As compared with spectacle lenses that have Abbe numbers above 100, the values of common IOLs are much lower, and between 37 and 55. For IOLs, the Abbe number depends only on the refractive index of the material, being worse with high refractive indexes [29].

Posterior Capsule Opacification
The biocompatibility of IOL material is often reported as the ability to avoid posterior capsule opacification, and to delay the need for Nd:YAG laser posterior capsulotomy. Hydrophobic materials are not permeable to water, and therefore cell proliferation behind lens optics is somewhat delayed. Posterior capsule fibrosis was especially associated with silicone optics. Hydrophilic acrylic is water permeable, and therefore some cell nutrients may cross IOL optic, thus favoring Elschnig pearl formation. However, recent research clearly demonstrated that optics shape is more important than the optics material in preventing PCO. When the angle formed by the optic surface and the optic border is very sharp and square ('square edge' design), posterior capsule opacification is delayed regardless of the physical properties of the material itself [19]. The easiest way to the square edge design is to limit or avoid polishing, a process through which IOLs are refined after punching or lathing. To be effective, the square edge must be complete around 360° and even at the optic-haptic junction, an issue especially important with plate-haptic IOLs.

Optics

The optics of IOLs has more curved surfaces than spectacle lenses of the same power because they lay in aqueous humor which has a refractive index of 1.33. The shape of the optics can be meniscus, plano-convex or biconvex, as depicted in figure 12. Currently, the biconvex design is the most employed, with different relations between the anterior and the posterior curvature. Flatter anterior/steeper posterior lenses mimic the natural lens shape, but they have been associated with

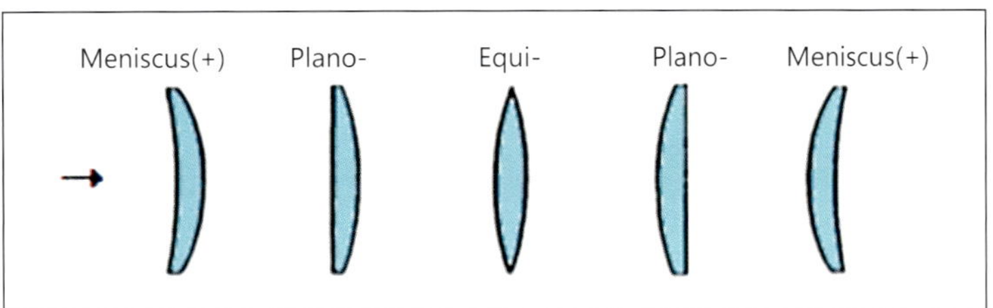

Fig. 12. Optics shapes available with current IOLs.

dysphotopsia, and currently are less popular than steeper anterior/flatter posterior or equiconvex design. The optics shape directly affects the position of the principal planes of IOLs, the two conjugated planes that define the optical properties of the lens, and the position on the visual axis of the principal points (and also nodal points because the refractive index of aqueous and vitreous is roughly the same), where the optical power of the lens is applied. Meniscus lenses have the nodal points outside the optics, plano-convex lenses have one at the lens surface, biconvex lenses have both within the optics, and nearer the more curved surface (fig. 13). For a given IOL power, the effective power in the implanted eye will depend on the position of the principal planes and points, therefore on lens shape and haptics vaulting. These properties are summarized by the 'A' constant, a number associated with every IOL that usually is between 117 and 120 for posterior chamber lenses. The 'A' constant comes from the old SRK I formula for IOL power calculation [30], a regression formula based on statistics that is reported here for reference only:

IOL power (dpt) = A constant – 0.9 mean K (dpt) – 2.5 axial length (mm)

The SRK I formula is no longer used because more accurate formulas are now available for precise IOL power calculation, but the 'A' constant is still employed worldwide to characterize the position of the principal planes of the IOL, and to anticipate the effective lens position after implantation. So, if our calculation indicates +22-dpt lens

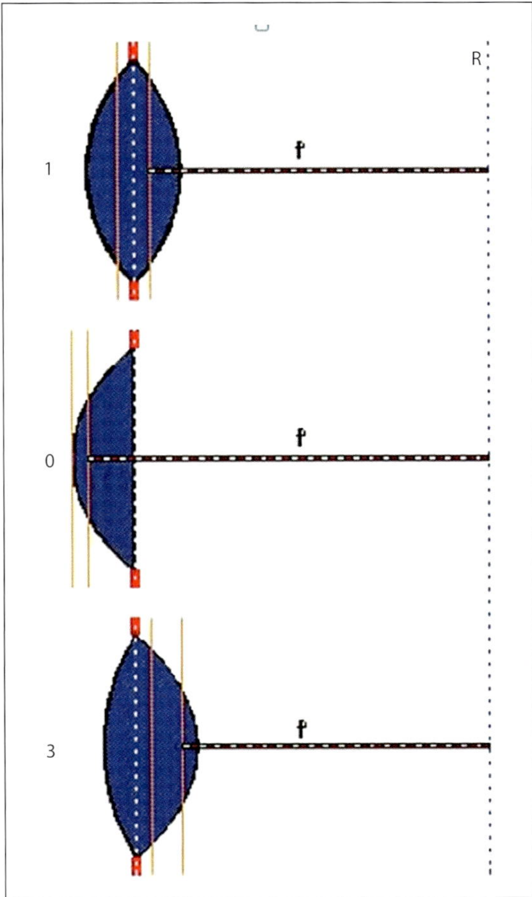

Fig. 13. Principal planes vs. optics shape.

power for 'A' = 118.2, this means +22.5 if the constant of the selected IOL is 118.7, and +23.5 if the constant of our lens is 119.7. We are recommended to verify our refractive results, and personalizing the constant for our area.

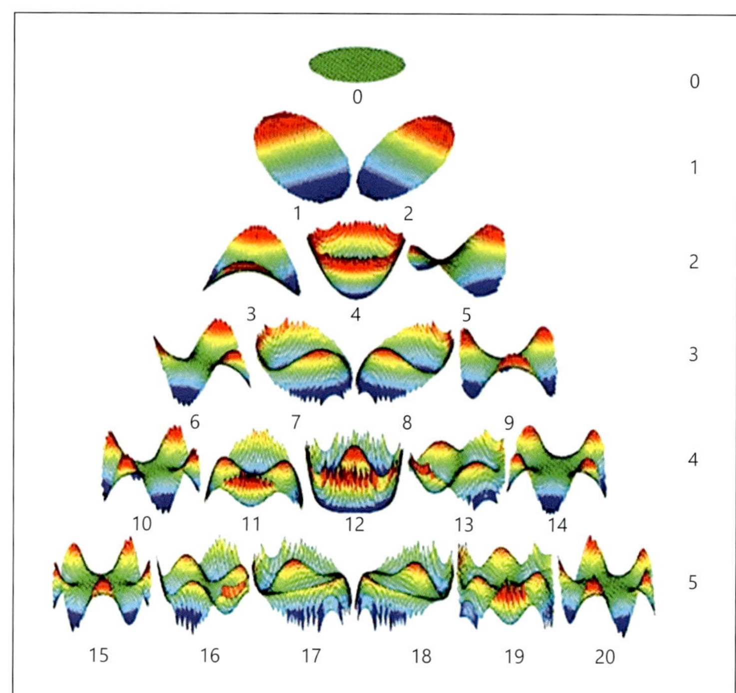

Fig. 14. Zernicke's decomposition of optical aberrations. The numbers on the right represent the aberration order.

Intraocular Lens Power Calculation

For every eye, IOL power is calculated according to several available formulas that are incorporated in any measuring device. The several available formulas can be simple corrections of the old SRK I, or complex calculations taking into account a number of parameters. The simplest formulas only require axial length and keratometry for power calculation. Anterior chamber depth comes next, with corneal diameter and thickness, and posterior lens capsule position as further parameters sometimes required. Recently, ultrasound instruments to measure axial length have been replaced by laser interferometry for increased precision. Optical formulas are better than regression formulas in long or short eyes, but even the most accurate calculation can end up with a refractive surprise, and we must be cautious in promising the abandon of glasses to patients. The most inaccurate results are obtained in eyes with previous corneal surgeries. These eyes require specific IOL power calculations, as the common formulas are not valid, usually leading to postoperative hyperopia in originally myopic eyes, and to postoperative myopia in originally hyperopic eyes.

Optical Aberration of the Normal and Pseudophakic Eye: Spherical and Aspheric Intraocular Lenses

By analyzing the refracted wavefront, we can define, study and quantify the optical aberration (= deviation from perfect image refraction) induced by any optical system, including the human eye. According to the popular Zernicke decomposition (fig. 14), optical aberrations are classified as low-order aberration – orders of 0 to 2 –, and high-order aberrations – orders of 3 and more [31].

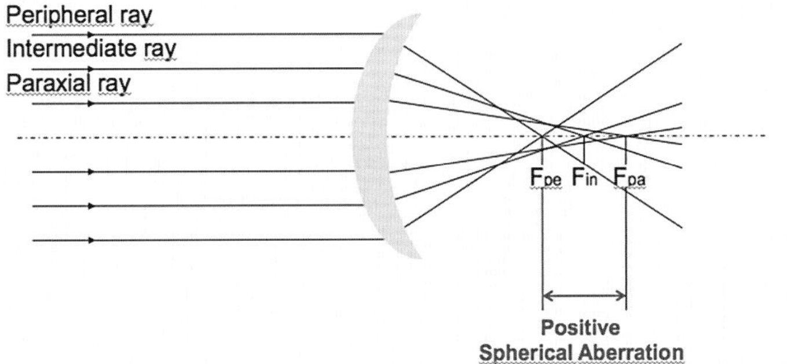

Fig. 15. Spherical aberration develops when peripheral rays and paraxial rays are refracted onto different foci.

Order 0 is a piston, i.e. the wavefront is perfectly reproduced but with delay as compared with the speed of light. Order 1 is a prism, i.e. the wavefront is perfect but tilted as compared to the incoming wavefront. Order 2 comprises spherical and astigmatic errors, those usually corrected by spectacle lenses. Order 3 is a combination of vertical and horizontal coma, and of trefoil. Order 4 deals with spherical aberration, second astigmatism and quadrafoil. Order 5 is again coma, order 6 again spherical aberration and so on.

After correcting for the low order with appropriate spectacles, the most important aberrations in clinical practice are: vertical coma Z3 (–1), horizontal coma Z3 (+1), and spherical aberration Z4 (0) [32]. Coma is the aberration of keratoconus, and gives a sort of tail to one side of the refracted image. Spherical aberration is the aberration of any spherical lens, moving the focus of peripheral rays towards the lens itself ('positive spherical aberration') or opposite the lens itself ('negative spherical aberration'; fig. 15). It should be noted that the human cornea has positive spherical aberration and a very low amount of coma. In the young, this positive spherical aberration is balanced by the natural human lens.

With aging, the balance is lost because of lens changes, and the old eye develops positive spherical aberration [33].

Spherical and Aspheric Intraocular Lens Design
The first design adopted for IOLs was the simple spherical design. Both engineers and ophthalmologists were aware that this design was far from optimal as it would add positive spherical aberration to that of the cornea, thus producing a highly aberrated optical system [34]. However, there was no way to ensure optic centration after IOL implantation, and therefore aspheric lenses that might correct spherical aberration were judged worse than spherical [35]. With the advent of capsular bag implantation, the idea came back to use IOL optics to correct the positive spherical aberration of the cornea, thus reproducing the condition of the young eye [36]. In pseudophakic eyes, spherical aberration has two main components: (1) the spherical aberration of the corneal surface, usually +0.3 at 6-mm optical zone, that shows little variation with individuals and age and is compensated by the natural lens in the young eye, and (2) the spherical aberration induced by the lens itself, usually positive, that varies with the diop-

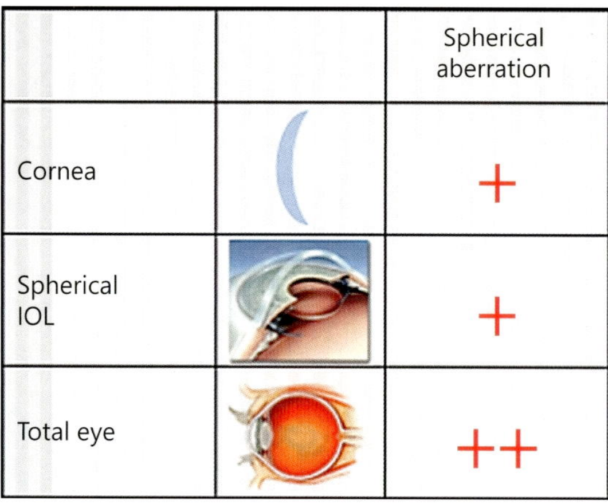

		Spherical aberration
Cornea		+
Spherical IOL		+
Total eye		++

Fig. 16. Spherical aberration is positive on the cornea, and positive on spherical IOLs.

tric power (fig. 16). Aspheric IOL design tries to correct for one or both of these components of spherical aberration [37].

The 'aberration-correcting' design attempts to correct for both IOL-induced and corneal spherical aberration, to produce a pseudophakic eye with virtually zero spherical aberration [36]. This is obtained by incorporating a highly prolate aspheric profile with 'negative' spherical aberration onto the anterior (AMO Tecnis) or the posterior optics surface. It should be noted that these lenses should be considered 'hyperaspheric' as they are not truly aspheric: they are given an optical defect – negative spherical aberration – to balance an opposite defect laying on the corneal surface.

Differently, the 'aberration-free' design attempts to correct only for the IOL-induced spherical aberration, to produce a pseudophakic eye whose spherical aberration is equal to that of the corneal surface [38]. This is obtained by incorporating a prolate aspheric design onto one of the two optic surfaces. Currently, this approach is represented by the Bausch & Lomb Advanced Optics IOLs. The claimed advantage of this approach is the ability to fit every eye, even those with corneal low positive or negative spherical aberration.

A third approach takes into account the low positive spherical aberration shown by some eyes with 'supernormal' visual acuity, and aims at producing pseudophakic eyes with amounts of spherical aberration that are intermediate between those obtained with the two previous designs [39]. Several companies are following this concept, including Alcon with the WF series [40].

Effect of Aspheric Lenses on Spherical Aberration
The efficacy of aspheric lenses in compensating for spherical aberration has been demonstrated in implanted eyes by means of aberrometers (fig. 17, 18) [41]. The refractive effect of this reduction in spherical aberration is the lack of refraction shift occurring with mydriasis. By comparing the 4-mm and 6-mm refractions, we found a myopic shift of –0.08 dpt with the Tecnis IOL, and of –0.57 to –0.90 dpt with conventional IOLs (p < 0.01) [41].

The effects of this aberration correction on the optical quality of the eyes can be devised from the Strehl ratio, an indicator of the point spread function (PSF) [42]. The eyes implanted with the aspheric version showed better results than those that had received the parent spherical IOL (fig. 19). The same pattern of improved values with the aspheric lens was observed for the modulation transfer function (MTF; fig. 20) [43].

The contrast sensitivity function is the subjective counterpart of the MTF, and therefore it is expected to improve following aspheric IOL implantation. Macular contrast sensitivity has been extensively studied with the Tecnis aspheric IOL, in comparison with different types of conventional IOLs [44, 45]. Most studies found better contrast sensitivity for the aspheric lens, although with different patterns. This improvement in contrast sensitivity has been associated with the improvement in night driving efficiency measured by driving simulators in some studies [46]: a fact that could better be related to the improved appreciation of peripheral targets due to the lack of night myopia.

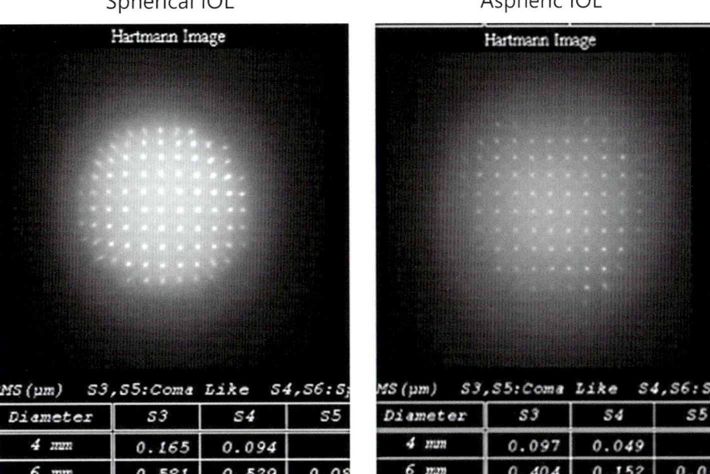

Diameter	S3	S4	S5
4 mm	0.165	0.094	
6 mm	0.581	0.529	0.08

Diameter	S3	S4	S5
4 mm	0.097	0.049	
6 mm	0.404	0.152	0.05

Fig. 17. Hartmann-Shack image of the wavefront with spherical and aspheric IOLs.

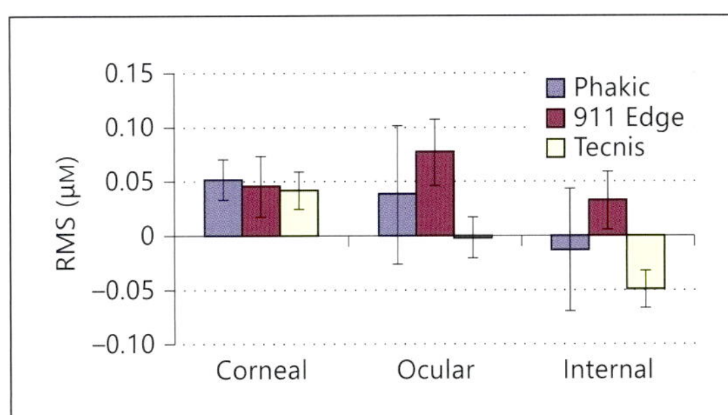

Fig. 18. Compensation of corneal spherical aberration by aspheric IOLs. Sphere Z4 (0), 4-mm optical zone. RMS = root mean square.

Inconveniences of Aspheric Intraocular Lenses

With all the aspheric IOLs, the improvements of the total wavefront aberration and of the PSF measured in the implanted eyes are less than optimal [47]. In addition, many eyes show an increase in coma that could explain these lower-than-expected improvements [48]. These drawbacks could be related to not yet clarified questions concerning current wavefront IOLs.

According to physical optics, the actual amount of spherical aberration to be corrected varies with the total refractive power of the eye and with the position of the principal planes of the IOL within the eye itself. Therefore, it is difficult for a +22 dpt lens with a given amount of asphericity to compensate for the spherical aberration in eyes with different corneal powers and IOL positions.

Because the dioptric power varies with eccentricity, aspheric IOLs are very sensitive to decentration and tilt. Even low degrees of decentration or tilt induce significant amounts of coma with the loss of advantages in terms of total aberration and optical quality, even though the effect on spherical aberration is maintained. It has been demonstrated on optical benches that the more aspheric the IOL, the more sensitive it is to decentration [49].

In addition, from a clinical point of view, the depth of focus is reduced with aspheric IOLs because of the correction of spherical aberration. This may be the reason why not all the published studies found aspheric IOLs definitely better than spherical in clinical practice [50].

Despite these inconveniences, aspheric IOLs are increasingly popular, and many IOLs are produced only with the aspheric profile. For the best result, we should select the proper IOL aspheric-

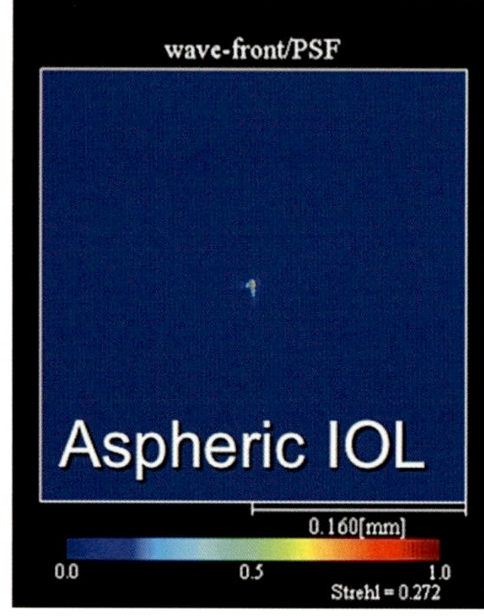

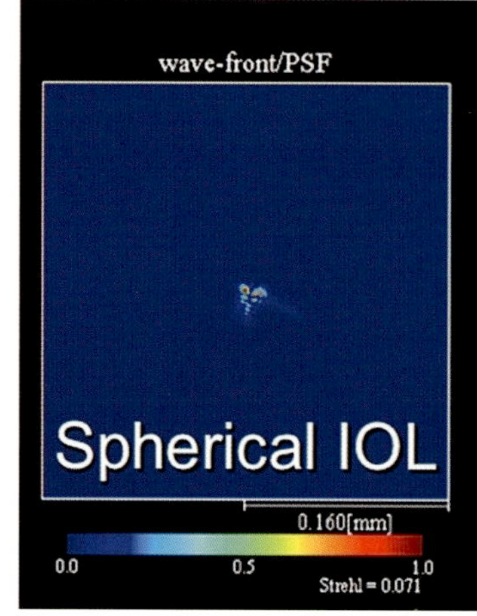

Fig. 19. PSF with spherical and aspheric IOLs.

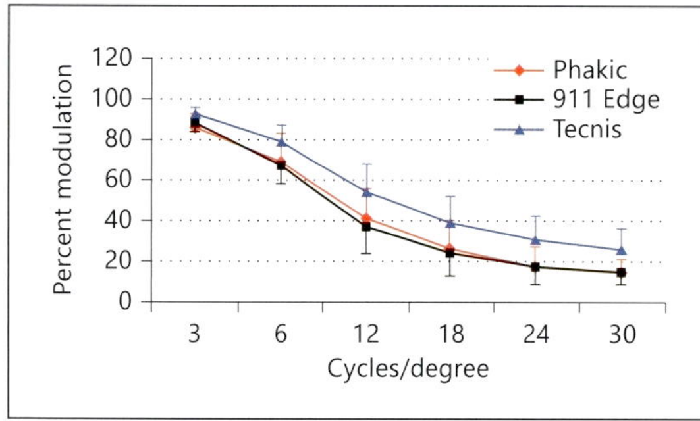

Fig. 20. MTF (4-mm optical zone) with spherical and aspheric IOLs.

ity according to the preoperative corneal spherical aberration, a value we can obtain with every corneal topographer [37].

Optics Design: Toric and Multifocal

Toric IOLs are now available to correct corneal astigmatism, and have been proven effective in clinical trials [51, 52]. The toricity can be incorporated in the anterior or posterior surface, or divided into the two. There are several sites on the Web to help surgeons in power calculation, both for the sphere and for the cylinder, also offering personalized IOLs in some instances. Results will depend on the accuracy of alignment. Every degree of misalignment will produce a 3% reduction of the effect, and above 30° the eventual astigmatism will be greater than the preoperative corneal astigmatism [53]. For this reason, IOLs that show the ability to rotate after implantation cannot be used as platforms for toric design.

Multifocal IOLs have been available for 25 years, and have never entered into wide clinical practice. They will be treated separately. Recently, toric multifocal IOLs have also become available.

Light Scattering and Optical Quality

Optical aberrations are produced by deviations of the light rays from their intended path, and their measurement gives no information about other important features of image transmission by any optical system, eye included. Light scattering and transparency of the media cannot be measured with a Hartmann-Shack aberrometer as it does not take into account the light that enters the eye and is therefore called a 'single-pass' device. To measure light scattering and the attenuation the light

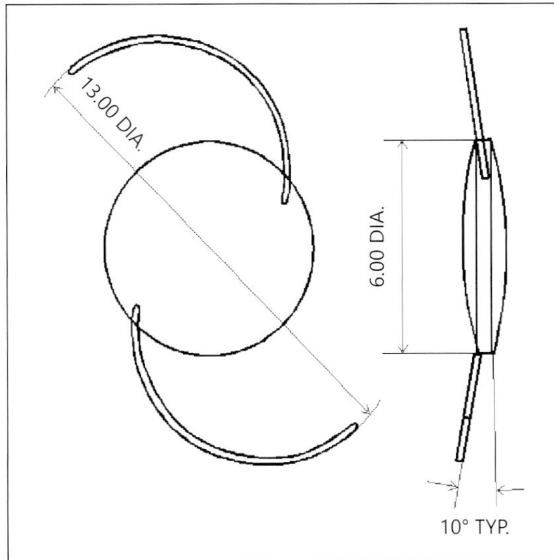

Fig. 21. Angulated IOL haptics.

undergoes while passing the optical system of the eye, we need a 'double-pass' instrument [54]. There are a few models available, the OQAS system being probably the most popular [55]. These devices can give information about the actual optical quality in implanted eyes, but their sensitivity even to the mildest PCO allows lens comparison only intraindividually to have the same cornea, and after laser posterior capsulotomy.

Haptics

The haptics are an important part of any IOL, often contributing to success or failure, and must be considered carefully to avoid mistakes and postoperative problems. The ability of the IOL to incorporate complex optics like multifocal, toric, and toric multifocal depends on the stability of the IOL after implantation, i.e. on the IOL haptics.

Three-Piece Intraocular Lens
In 3-piece IOLs, the haptics have the form of a 'C' (C-loop IOLs), and are usually inserted into two holes prepared in the optic border. They may form an angle with the lens plane, usually 5–10°, to avoid iris capture when the lens is sulcus implanted (fig. 21). Three-piece IOLs are less popular today because at implantation they require a larger incision than 1-piece IOL, and are especially used for sulcus implantation after posterior capsule rupture. Three-piece IOLs are preferred in infants [56] as it is easier to implant the loops in the ciliary sulcus, and the optics behind the posterior capsule after posterior capsulorhexis. It should be noted that PMMA IOLs do have C-loop haptics, but they are usually single piece. The ability of the C-loop haptics to keep the capsular bag round without ovalizing it is considered an advantage. Unfortunately, long loops are difficult to manage at implantation, and cannot be injected as shorter loops are.

Originally, the haptics were made of 4/0 or 5/0 polypropylene, but this material was abandoned because of postoperative degradation inside the eye. Nowadays, they are commonly made of three materials: PMMA, PVDF, and polyammide.

PMMA haptics are fragile unless a compression molding production was adopted. Even so, they can be bent at implantation and show low memory leading to optic decentration [57]. This can be especially harmful with silicone optics that forms no adherence to the lens capsule. Silicone IOLs with PMMA haptics are no longer preferred for sulcus implantation. After bag placement, PMMA loops can be compressed towards the optics by bag contraction forces, causing some IOL decentration, especially with eccentric capsulorhexis.

PVDF is a chemical compound with better memory and better flexibility than PMMA [58]. It is a better material for haptics, and obtains a strong adhesion with the lens capsule after bag placement. However, it is almost impossible to remove it after capsule sealing.

Polyamide is employed for haptics by some companies. It is a very flexible material, and its location behind the iris might prevent degradation. The process of capsule sealing will maintain the IOL optics in place even if the haptics undergo degradation; however, silicone optics might dislocate into the vitreous chamber through a wide posterior capsulotomy.

Single-Piece IOL

Single-piece IOLs include a variety of models and materials. There are models with C-loops designed for sulcus and bag implantation, made of rigid and foldable acrylic, both hydrophobic and hydrophilic, that are similar to 3-piece IOLs as for IOL selection and implantation (fig. 22). There are shorter models specifically designed for bag implantation made of hydrophobic acrylic material. Some of these lenses have 2 haptics in the form of a modified C-loop (fig. 22); others have 3, 4, or 6 haptics in the attempt to resist posterior pressure and capsular bag contraction without being displaced. A popular design is the plate-haptic lens (fig. 23), especially for toric models because they allow clockwise and counterclockwise rotation. However, plate-haptic silicone lenses can be 'squeezed' into the vitreous chamber by capsular bag contraction after laser posterior capsulotomy.

Currently, short and thin single-piece hydrophilic IOLs are used after MICS because they can be implanted through a 1.7-mm incision. Research is ongoing looking for better injectors that could deliver even hydrophobic single-piece IOLs through sub-2-mm incisions.

Anterior Chamber Lenses

Angle-supported IOLs are available in rigid and foldable hydrophobic acrylic material (fig. 24) to be implanted after complicated cataract surgery or in phakic eyes for refractive purposes. IOL sizing is crucial, and IOL length should exceed the anterior chamber diameter by 0.5 mm. Their use is controversial as endothelial and iris damage has been reported at intervals for almost all models.

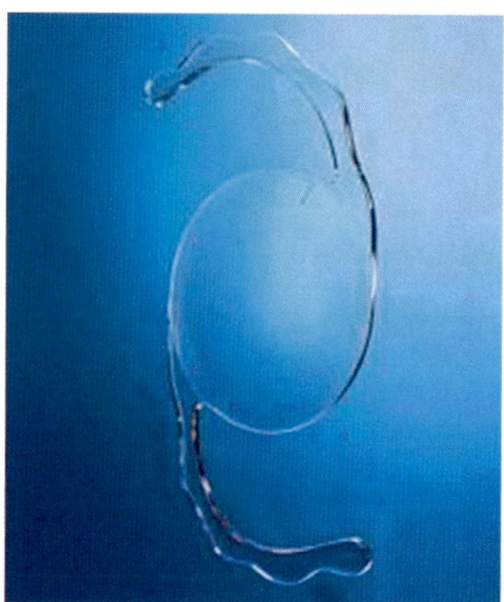

Fig. 22. Foldable hydrophilic acrylic IOL for sulcus placement.

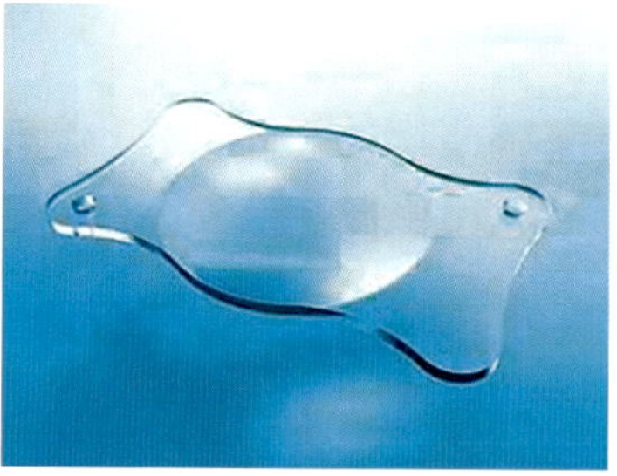

Fig. 23. Plate-haptic hydrophilic acrylic IOL.

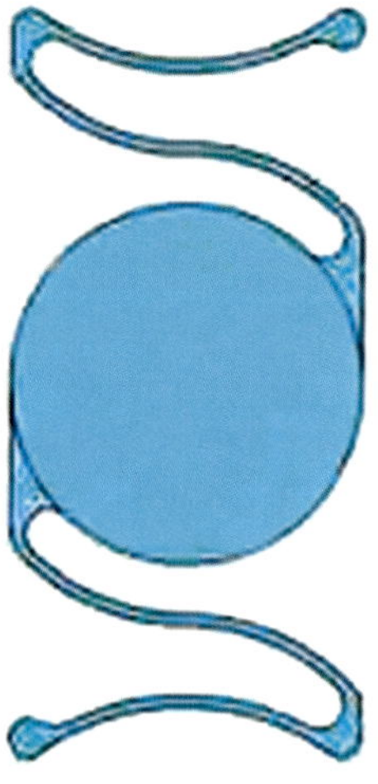

Fig. 24. Anterior chamber angle-supported IOL.

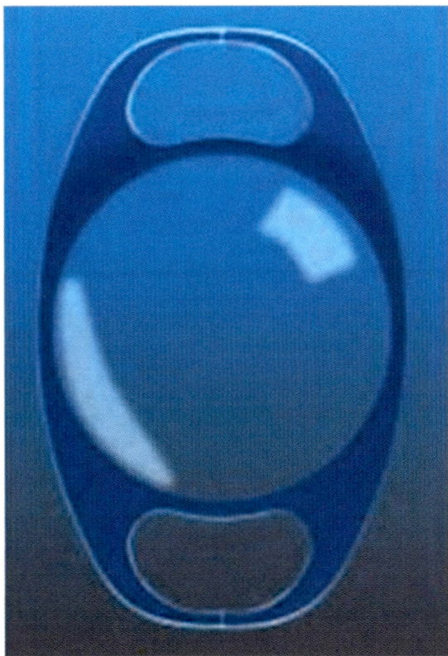

Fig. 25. IOL for iris fixation.

Iris-claw lenses have been available since the 1970s, and are still employed with success in aphakic and phakic eyes. The models differ slightly (fig. 25), and have the advantage of 'one size fits all'. Aphakic iris claw lenses can be implanted behind the iris, taking into account the 'A' constant change.

Posterior Chamber Phakic Intraocular Lenses

The VIsian ICL (STAAR Surgical, Monrovia, Calif., USA) is a plate haptic lens made of Collamer designed to be implanted over the natural lens behind the iris. It will be discussed in the dedicated chapter.

Intraocular Telescopes

Special attempts have been made to address the problem of age-related macular degeneration. The current implantable mirror telescope (LMI, Optolight, Israel) is a thick IOL that provides image magnification and can help retinas with dry macular degeneration in reading. In selected eyes, the improvement in visual acuity was as high as 30 ETDRS letters, according to published results.

Disclosure Statement

The author is a consultant for Bausch & Lomb, and has received research grants from Hanita Lenses, Acritec-Zeiss, and SIFI.

References

These references are only a small part of the huge literature about IOLs. They may be used as a guide to help further research.

1 Ridley H: Intraocular acrylic lenses – past, present and future. Trans Ophthalmol Soc UK 1964;84:5–14.
2 Shearing S: A practical posterior chamber lens. CLAO J 1978;4:114–117.
3 Ram J, Gupta N, Sukhija JS, Chaudhary M, Verma N, Kumar S, Severia S: Outcome of cataract surgery with primary intraocular lens implantation in children. Br J Ophthalmol 2011;95:1086–1090.
4 Michelson J, Werner L, Ollerton A, Leishman L, Bodnar Z: Light scattering and light transmittance in intraocular lenses explanted because of optic opacification. J Cataract Refract Surg 2012;38:1476–1485.
5 Mazzocco TR, Rajacich GM, Epstein E: Soft Implant Lenses in Cataract Surgery. Slack, Thorofare, 1986.
6 Baillif S, Ecochard R, Hartmann D, Freney J, Kodjikian L: Intraocular lens and cataract surgery: comparison between bacterial adhesion and risk of postoperative endophthalmitis according to intraocular lens biomaterial (in French). J Fr Ophtalmol 2009;32:515–528.
7 von Mohrenfels CW, Salgado J, Khoramnia R, Maier M, Lohmann CP: Clinical results with the light adjustable intraocular lens after cataract surgery. J Refract Surg 2010;26:314–320.
8 Hengerer FH, Hütz WW, Dick HB, Conrad-Hengerer I: Combined correction of axial hyperopia and astigmatism using the light adjustable intraocular lens. Ophthalmology 2011;118:1236–1241.
9 Rønbeck M, Behndig A, Taube M, Koivula A, Kugelberg M: Comparison of glistenings in intraocular lenses with three different materials: 12-year follow-up. Acta Ophthalmol 2013;91:66–70.
10 Bartz-Schmidt KU, Konen W, Esser P, Walter P, Heimann K: Intraocular silicone lenses and silicone oil (in German). Klin Monbl Augenheilkd 1995;207:162–166.
11 Cunanan CM, Ghazizadeh M, Buchen SY, Knight PM: Contact-angle analysis of intraocular lenses. J Cataract Refract Surg 1998;24:341–351.

12 Oshika T, Shiokawa Y: Effect of folding on the optical quality of soft acrylic intraocular lenses. J Cataract Refract Surg 1996;22(suppl 2):1360–1364.

13 Radford SW, Carlsson AM, Barrett GD: Comparison of pseudophakic dysphotopsia with Akreos Adapt and SN60-AT intraocular lenses. J Cataract Refract Surg 2007;33:88–93.

14 Bournas P, Drazinos S, Kanellas D, Arvanitis M, Vaikoussis E: Dysphotopsia after cataract surgery: comparison of four different intraocular lenses. Ophthalmologica 2007;221:378–383.

15 Miura M, Osako M, Elsner AE, Kajizuka H, Yamada K, Usui M: Birefringence of intraocular lenses. J Cataract Refract Surg 2004;30:1549–1555.

16 Ollerton A, Werner L, Fuller SR, Kavoussi SC, McIntyre JS, Mamalis N: Evaluation of a new single-piece 4% water content hydrophobic acrylic intraocular lens in the rabbit model. J Cataract Refract Surg 2012;38:1827–1832.

17 Chehade M, Elder MJ: Intraocular lens materials and styles: a review. Aust N Z J Ophthalmol 1997;25:255–263.

18 Kohnen T, Klaproth OK: Intraocular lenses for microincisional cataract surgery (in German). Ophthalmologe 2010;107:127–135.

19 Hazra S, Palui H, Vemuganti GK: Comparison of design of intraocular lens versus the material for PCO prevention. Int J Ophthalmol 2012;5:59–63.

20 Gimbel HV, Condon GP, Kohnen T, Olson RJ, Halkiadakis I: Late in-the-bag intraocular lens dislocation: incidence, prevention, and management. J Cataract Refract Surg 2005;31:2193–2204.

21 Apple DJ, Werner L: Complications of cataract and refractive surgery: a clinicopathological documentation. Trans Am Ophthalmol Soc 2001;99:95–109.

22 Trivedi RH, Werner L, Apple DJ, Pandey SK, Izak AM: Post cataract-intraocular lens (IOL) surgery opacification. Eye 2002;16:217–241.

23 Brown DC, Ziémba SL: Collamer intraocular lens: clinical results from the US FDA core study. J Cataract Refract Surg 2001;27:833–840.

24 Schild G, Amon M, Abela-Formanek C, Schauersberger J, Bartl G, Kruger A: Uveal and capsular biocompatibility of a single-piece, sharp-edged hydrophilic acrylic intraocular lens with collagen (Collamer): 1-year results. J Cataract Refract Surg 2004;30:1254–1258.

25 Lombardo M, De Santo MP, Lombardo G, Barberi R, Serrao S: Analysis of intraocular lens surface properties with atomic force microscopy. J Cataract Refract Surg 2006;32:1378–1384.

26 Welch NR, Gregori N, Zabriskie N, Olson RJ: Satisfaction and dysphotopsia in the pseudophakic patient. Can J Ophthalmol 2010;45:140–143.

27 Kontadakis GA, Plainis S, Moschandreas J, Tsika C, Pallikaris IG, Tsilimbaris MK: In vivo evaluation of blue-light attenuation with tinted and untinted intraocular lenses. J Cataract Refract Surg 2011;37:1031–1037.

28 Lindstrom RL, Doddi N: Ultraviolet light absorption in intraocular lenses. J Cataract Refract Surg 1986;12:285–289.

29 Zhao H, Mainster MA: The effect of chromatic dispersion on pseudophakic optical performance. Br J Ophthalmol 2007;91:1225–1229.

30 Sanders D, Retzlaff J, Kraff M, Kratz R, Gills J, Levine R, Colvard M, Weisel J, Loyd T: Comparison of the accuracy of the Binkhorst, Colenbrander, and SRK implant power prediction formulas. J Am Intraocul Implant Soc 1981;7:337–340.

31 Kuroda T, Fujikado T, Maeda N, Oshika T, Hirohara Y, Mihashi T: Wavefront analysis of higher-order aberrations in patients with cataract. J Cataract Refract Surg 2002;28:438–444.

32 Applegate RA, Howland HC: Refractive surgery, optical aberrations, and visual performance. J Refract Surg 1997;13:295–299.

33 Williams D, Yoon GY, Porter J, Guirao A, Hofer H, Cox I: Visual benefit of correcting higher order aberrations of the eye. J Refract Surg 2000;16:S554–S559.

34 Uchio E, Ohno S, Kusakawa T: Spherical aberration and glare disability with intraocular lenses of different optical design. J Cataract Refract Surg 1995;21:690–696.

35 Atchison DA: Design of aspheric intraocular lenses. Ophthalmic Physiol Opt 1991;11:137–146.

36 Holladay JT, Piers PA, Koranyi G, van der Mooren M, Norrby NE: A new intraocular lens design to reduce spherical aberration of pseudophakic eyes. J Refract Surg 2002;18:683–691.

37 Bellucci R, Morselli S: Optimizing higher-order aberrations with intraocular lens technology. Curr Opin Ophthalmol 2007;18:67–73.

38 Altmann GE, Nichamin LD, Lane SS, Pepose JS: Optical performance of 3 intraocular lens designs in the presence of decentration. J Cataract Refract Surg 2005;31:574–585.

39 Lombardo M, Lombardo G: Wave aberration of human eyes and new descriptors of image optical quality and visual performance. J Cataract Refract Surg 2010;36:313–331.

40 Tzelikis PF, Akaishi L, Trindade FC, Boteon JE: Ocular aberrations and contrast sensitivity after cataract surgery with AcrySof IQ intraocular lens implantation: clinical comparative study. J Cataract Refract Surg 2007;33:1918–1924.

41 Bellucci R, Morselli S, Piers P: Comparison of wavefront aberrations and optical quality of eyes implanted with five different intraocular lenses. J Refract Surg 2004;20:297–306.

42 Pieh S, Fiala W, Malz A, Stork W: In vitro strehl ratios with spherical, aberration-free, average, and customized spherical aberration-correcting intraocular lenses. Invest Ophthalmol Vis Sci 2009;50:1264–1270.

43 Rawer R, Stork W, Spraul CW, Lingenfelder C: Imaging quality of intraocular lenses. J Cataract Refract Surg 2005;31:1618–1631.

44 Montés-Micó R, Ferrer-Blasco T, Cerviño A: Analysis of the possible benefits of aspheric intraocular lenses: review of the literature. J Cataract Refract Surg 2009;35:172–181.

45 Dick HB: Recent developments in aspheric intraocular lenses. Curr Opin Ophthalmol 2009;20:25–32.

46 Denoyer A, Denoyer L, Halfon J, Majzoub S, Pisella PJ: Comparative study of aspheric intraocular lenses with negative spherical aberration or no aberration. J Cataract Refract Surg 2009;35:496–503.

47 Gong XH, Zheng QX, Wang N, Chen D, Zhao J, Li J, Zhao YE: Visual and optical performance of eyes with different corneal spherical aberration implanted with aspheric intraocular lens. Int J Ophthalmol 2012;5:323–328.

48 Bellucci R, Morselli S, Pucci V: Spherical aberration and coma with an aspherical and a spherical intraocular lens in normal age-matched eyes. J Cataract Refract Surg 2007;33:203–209.

49 Sauer T, Mester U: Tilt and decentration of an intraocular lens implanted in the ciliary sulcus after capsular bag defect during cataract surgery. Graefes Arch Clin Exp Ophthalmol 2013;251:89–93.

50 Morales EL, Rocha KM, Chalita MR, Nosé W, Avila MP: Comparison of optical aberrations and contrast sensitivity between aspheric and spherical intraocular lenses. J Refract Surg 2011;27:723–728.

51 Langenbucher A, Viestenz A, Szentmáry N, Behrens-Baumann W, Viestenz A: Toric intraocular lenses – theory, matrix calculations, and clinical practice. J Refract Surg 2009;25:611–622.

52 Ahmed II, Rocha G, Slomovic AR, Climenhaga H, Gohill J, Grégoire A, Ma J: Visual function and patient experience after bilateral implantation of toric intraocular lenses. J Cataract Refract Surg 2010;36:609–616.

53 Jin H, Limberger IJ, Ehmer A, Guo H, Auffarth GU: Impact of axis misalignment of toric intraocular lenses on refractive outcomes after cataract surgery. J Cataract Refract Surg 2010;36:2061–2072.

54 Nam J, Thibos LN, Bradley A, Himebaugh N, Liu H: Forward light scatter analysis of the eye in a spatially-resolved double-pass optical system. Opt Express 2011;19:7417–7438.

55 Vilaseca M, Peris E, Pujol J, Borras R, Arjona M: Intra- and intersession repeatability of a double-pass instrument. Optom Vis Sci 2010;87:675–681.

56 Faramarzi A, Javadi MA: Comparison of 2 techniques of intraocular lens implantation in pediatric cataract surgery. J Cataract Refract Surg 2009;35:1040–1045.

57 Lane SS, Burgi P, Milios GS, Orchowski MW, Vaughan M, Schwarte E: Comparison of the biomechanical behavior of foldable intraocular lenses. J Cataract Refract Surg 2004;30:2397–2402.

58 Izak AM, Werner L, Apple DJ, Macky TA, Trivedi RH, Pandey SK: Loop memory of haptic materials in posterior chamber intraocular lenses. J Cataract Refract Surg 2002;28:1229–1235.

Roberto Bellucci, MD
Ophthalmic Unit, Department of Neurosciences
Hospital and University of Verona, Borgo Trento Hospital
IT–37126 Verona (Italy)
E-Mail roberto.bellucci@ospedaleuniverona.it

Güell JL (ed): Cataract. ESASO Course Series. Basel, Karger, 2013, vol 3, pp 56–61
DOI: 10.1159/000350906

Femtolaser Cataract Surgery

Zoltan Z. Nagy

Department of Ophthalmology, Semmelweis University, Budapest, Hungary

Abstract

In recent years femtosecond laser cataract surgery has been an accepted procedure in cataract surgery. In this book chapter the technical aspects of the femtosecond laser systems will be discussed. The most important indications and contraindications of femtolaser cataract surgery will be also described in details. Surgeons might encounter findings during and following femtolaser treatment, which are different from traditional phacoemulsification. These might include subconjunctival redness, pupillary constriction, capsular blockage syndrome, wound incision difficulties. The chapter also discusses how to recognise and handle this problems. Besides of these, ergonomics and the suggested planned series of the procedures will be shown at the end.

Various lasers (light amplification by stimulated emission of radiation) have been used in ophthalmology for more than 50 years. Ophthalmology always had a pioneering role in laser use. All lasers operate at a specific wavelength, pulse pattern, pulse energy, pulse duration, repetition rate and spot size. According to these parameters, they are absorbed in different tissues at different length, and the biological effect also varies. Today, there is no tissue within the eye which could not be treated with some type of laser. Many lasers operate with the local thermal effect like photocoagulation (e.g. argon laser), others with photoablation (e.g. excimer lasers), or photodisruption (e.g.:YAG laser).

Interestingly, the Nd:YAG (neodymium-doped yttrium aluminum garnet) lasers and femtosecond lasers operate at similar wavelengths. On the other hand, the tissue effect is very different, because femtosecond lasers operate with extremely short duration of each pulse. The femtosecond time is in one quadrillionth, or 10^{-15} of a second, while Nd:YAG laser pulse duration is in the nanosecond range, i.e. 10^{-9}.

Femtosecond lasers appeared first in corneal surgery to create the corneal flap for refractive surgeons. Thereafter, the indication has been widened for all kinds of corneal surgery: lamellar and penetrating keratoplasty, segment implantation in keratoconus and pocket creation for presbyopia inlay treatments. The first corneal femtolasers operated at 30 kHz; then, the repetition rate was doubled. The latest 150-kHz femtolasers are able to create a corneal flap within 10 s. The higher the repetition rate, the lower the energy is required to obtain the same tissue effect.

Femtosecond lasers in cataract surgery use a pulse duration of 400–800 fs, the energy range is in microjoule, which is usually less than in YAG capsulotomy when the surgeon is using 1–3 µJ. During the surgery of the crystalline lens, femtosecond laser energy can be increased maximally to 10–15 µJ.

A photodisruption effect is achieved when the sharply focused beam of femtosecond duration has generated plasma within the affected tissue. The plasma expands at high speed in a shock wave form and displaces the surrounding tissues. With time, the plasma cools down, and so called cavitation bubbles are formed. At the tissue level, photodisruption occurs within the laser's focal point without any heat development or damage in the collateral tissues.

Based on the photodisruption principle, femtolaser for cataract surgery can create tissue separation and very precise cuts within the cornea, the lens capsule and within the crystalline lens.

The numerical aperture of different femtolasers is a very important characteristic in cornea and lens treatment. Numerical aperture affects significantly the spot size and volume. Higher numerical aperture results in less dispersion in the laser beam (better focused laser beam), and lower energy is needed to provide the same effect; the precision of the deep cut is also better. Therefore, corneal treatments need a higher numerical aperture and lower energy, while the crystalline lens needs a low numerical aperture with higher energy level. Femtosecond lasers can have a repetition rate up to 160 kHz. It is very important that a femtosecond laser treating the cornea and crystalline lens simultaneously have a great flexibility in pulse energy, pulse pattern, pulse duration and repetition rate.

Cataract surgery nowadays is the most frequently performed ophthalmic procedure. It is estimated that approximately 18 million cataract procedures are performed globally in a year, which will increase to 24 million very soon due to demographic changes, aging population and change in indication for lens surgery. Cataract surgery by now is not only a vision restoration procedure, but also a refractive type of operation. Ophthalmic surgeons do not only give back the clarity of the optical media, but freely change the refraction of the patients as well. Sometimes, patients have better vision quality after the lens procedure than before developing the cataract. Moreover, presbyopia treatment is also an option for patients and surgeons.

The exactness of refractive surgery is 10 times higher than that of cataract surgery; therefore, much progress still needs to be made. This is partly because during refractive procedures the patient has to bear the cost of the treatment, while cataract operation is usually covered by the insurance. Due to the fact that we have to operate on increasingly younger patients and the indication is not only pure cataract but a refractive error, presbyopia treatment, enhancement for previous refractive procedure, high myopia, high hyperopia, keratoconus, etc., patients are more demanding. A solution could reside in better lens planning and preoperative assessment. Another alternative is better surgical technique with more consistent results not depending on the dexterity only of the surgeon.

Regarding the surgical technique, femtolasers offer new potentials for patients and surgeons as well. The first ever human femtolaser-assisted cataract operation was performed in 2008 in the Department of Ophthalmology, Semmelweis University, Budapest, Hungary. The first experiences were reported in peer-reviewed ophthalmic journals [1–6].

Technical Aspects of the Alcon-LenSx Femtosecond Laser System

The Alcon-LenSx femtosecond laser operates with a solid-state laser source which produces thousands of femtosecond pulses per second. Laser pulses are delivered via a sophisticated beam delivery system to the eye. It includes an articulated arm, a series of different optical lenses, scanners and monitors. So far, the LenSx laser system utilizes uniquely a variable numerical aperture for optimal performance in both the corneal and the lens plane.

The first part of femtosecond surgery is the docking procedure, while the surgeon uses a curved contact lens which is integrated with a sterile limbal suction ring. The tubing uses a vacuum system for fixating the patient's eye. The patient interface is easy to dock, and it provides the largest viewing and surgical diameter range which allows performing the peripheral corneal wounds and arcuate keratotomy incisions. The patient interface usually elevates the intraocular pressure to not more than 35 mm Hg; therefore, ocular perfusion and visual perception are maintained during the femtolaser pretreatment.

The Alcon-LenSx femtolaser has a live video and proprietary HD OCT (optical coherence tomography) to help the docking and surgical pattern localization. The OCT uses the same optical path as the laser beam and is fully integrated and calibrated. The OCT covers the whole anterior segment up to the posterior capsule of the crystalline lens and is able to assess the lens density as well. The surgical pattern is automatically performed, the surgeon has the possibility to alter the automatically offered treatment parameters, such as centration of anterior capsulotomy, depth cut within the lens (distance from posterior and anterior capsule) and position of corneal cuts (fig. 1–3).

The OCT measurements effectively combine the circular and linear scans, which results in better depth and tilt information. The femtosecond laser produces a 100-μm shock wave; therefore, a minimum of 500-μm (rather 700-μm) safety distance is recommended from the posterior capsule.

Possible Surgical Findings after Femtolaser Treatment

Subconjunctival Redness or Hemorrhage
Mild to moderate redness and hemorrhages can be noted, especially in patients on anticoagulant therapy. In the case of proper preoperative consultation, patients readily accept this phenomenon. Redness usually resolves quickly.

Pupillary Constriction
Preoperatively, the pupil should be at least 6.0 mm in diameter. Shock waves from laser pulses can be close to the iris, especially in not well-dilated cases, which can cause inadvertent miosis. Preoperatively, more dilating agents are advised and also non-steroid anti-inflammatory drops (e.g. diclofenac). During laser programming, capsulotomy diameter should be at least 1.0 mm smaller than the pupillary diameter. The time between femtolaser pretreatment and cataract surgery should be as short as possible (5–10 min are recommended). In well-dilated normal cases, pretreatment of 2–3 patients is possible, but one femtolaser-one cataract surgery is the preferred pattern.

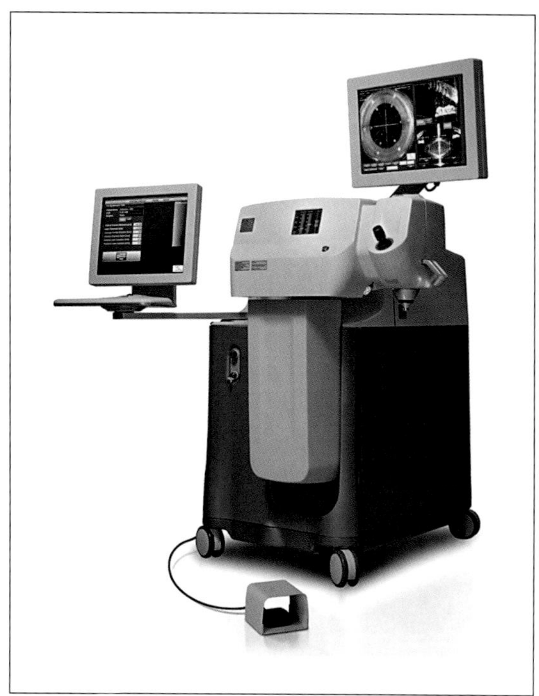

Fig. 1. The LenSx femtolaser.

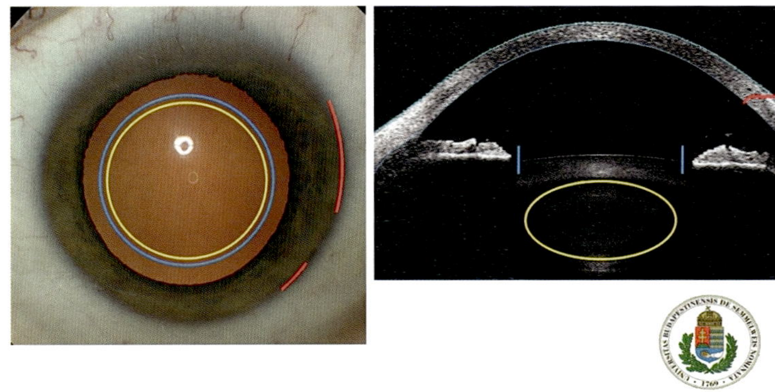

Fig. 2. Surgeon's screen. Note the corneal wounds and astigmatic incisions. In the right upper part, OCT identifies the endothelial layer and anterior capsule (highest and lowest point); in the lower part of the image, OCT identifies the cut within the crystalline lens (yellow area).

Fig. 3. The proprietary image-guided system allows the surgeon to take a preoperative OCT image and position the planned incisions and photolysis patterns on the patient's eye. The blue and yellow overlays represent lens photolysis and capsulotomy patterns. The red line represents corneal incisions. Size and position of all patterns can be preprogrammed and adjusted for ultimate control.

Capsular Blockage Syndrome

Intraoperative capsular blockage syndrome was first reported in 2011 during hydrodissection [7]. Large-diameter hydrodissection cannula with high-speed fluid egress may impede gas bubble to leave the nucleus. The consequent increase in pressure within the lens causes the rupture of the posterior capsule and sinking of the nucleus into the vitreous cavity. The so called 'rock-and-roll' technique helps to avoid this possible complication, i.e. after a meticulous, slow and gentle hydrodissection, the surgeon should gently press down (to 'rock') the nucleus and move it (to 'roll'). The suggested modification of the surgical technique (titrated injection of hydrodissection fluid and meticulous splitting of the nucleus) helps to release intralenticular gas bubble and to avoid this threatening complication.

Corneal Incision Sizing and Position

Femtolaser-created incision width may be tighter than expected; therefore, it is recommended to use the opening spatula and stretch with fine hand movements the edges of the incision. At programming, the surgeon should note the proper centration. In the case of decentration, corneal incisions are more central than expected, which might cause surgically induced astigmatism. Perfect docking is mandatory to avoid lens tilt and centrally shifted corneal incisions. In the latter case, lens capsulotomy and fragmentation might also be asymmetrical leading to partial capsulotomy and fragmentation.

Most Important Indications

The most important indications are as follows:
- Anterior capsulotomy.
- Laser fragmentation of the crystalline lens (harder lenses).
- Laser liquefaction of the crystalline lens (soft lenses).
- Single plane or multiplane (uniplanar, biplanar, triplanar, etc) corneal cuts with 2–3 incisions.
- Arcuate corneal cuts to control preoperative corneal astigmatism.

During femtolaser cataract surgery, the surgeon is able to modify all treatment parameters, e.g. he/she can change the diameter of capsulotomy to 4.5–6.0 mm (smaller diameter posterior chamber lens to accommodate lens requirements). Today, the so called hybrid pattern is recommended for lens fragmentation: the central 3.0-mm core is liquefied and the peripheral parts fragmented into 4–8 cuts (cross pattern and cake or pizza pattern). This pattern allows removing the central lens part easily and gives access to the peripheral parts, reducing the ultrasonic phacoenergy and time. This technique allows better visual acuity on the next postoperative day, reduced corneal edema and reduced cystoid macular edema. Among our patients, reduced retinal thickness was noted, presumably less phacoenergy due to femtolaser pretreatment. Additional benefits might be less manipulation within the eye thanks to the prefragmented nucleus. So far, lens fragmentation has been performed in all kinds of cataract, from soft to very hard lenses. Presently, it is recommended up to grade +4.0. In brunescent cataract, the water content of the crystalline lens is quite low; therefore, laser absorption is not perfect. On the other hand, in white tumescent cataracts the water content is very high; therefore, efficient lens fragmentation is very unlikely. In the latter cases, capsulotomy and corneal incisions provide the most important benefits of this technology.

Contraindications

There is only one contraindication, which is non-dilating pupil <6.0 mm in diameter. Capsulotomy is possible in the case of a central pupillary area 5.0 mm in diameter, but because the edge of the iris is within 1.0 mm, the chance of hitting the pupillary edge is high; the pupil might be narrower than expected at commencing phacoemulsification. Smaller capsulotomy can also be performed, but the chance of capsular phimosis is increased if the capsulotomy diameter is <4.0 mm.

Ergonomics

For the femtolaser equipment, a 11 × 14 ft (3.3 × 4.2 m) room dimension is recommended for ergonomic use. In the case of a larger room, the femtolaser can be placed into the same room as the phacoemulsification device.

Planned Series of Procedures

Capsulotomy should be performed first, then fragmentation/liquefaction and lastly corneal cuts. The reason behind it is that during lens fragmentation a gas bubble may appear within the lens, which might elevate the anterior capsule. If it occurs, another OCT measurement is required to redefine the treatment parameters; therefore, capsulotomy should be carried out first. Small gas bubbles freely move up to the endothelial layer, but this does not prevent effective lens fragmentation. Corneal cuts are performed lastly because they are performed from the inside to the outside. A previous gas bubble does not alter the anatomical parameters of the cornea.

In summary, the most important advantage of femtolaser cataract technology is that all steps can be customized, delivering unparalleled accuracy, repeatability and consistency in results. The fully integrated OCT imaging system, focus tracking and automated pattern prepositioning help and streamline the docking procedures and treatment planning. After docking, moderate suction is applied, the OCT swiftly scans the entire anterior segment and provides 3-D cross-sectional images from the anterior corneal surface until the posterior capsule. The surgeon should only confirm the prepositioned incisions or alter them. During treatment, the surgeon is able to follow the path of the laser beam on the LCD monitor. Treatment is initiated by pressing the foot pedal. Currently, the whole treatment time is between 40 and 60 s. After treatment completion, the suction is released, the curved patient interface is removed from the patient's eye, and cataract surgery combined with phacoemulsification may immediately begin.

References

1 Nagy ZZ, Takacs A, Filkorn T, Sarayba M: Initial clinical evaluation of intraocular femtosecond laser in cataract surgery. J Refract Surg 2009;25:1053–1060.
2 Nagy ZZ, Kranitz K, Takacs AI, Mihaltz K, Kovács I, Knorz MC, Nagy ZZ: Comparison of intraocular lens decentration parameters after femtosecond and manual capsulotomies. J Refract Surg 2011;27:564–569.
3 Kranitz K, Takacs A, Mihaltz K, Kovács I, Knorz MC, Nagy ZZ: Femtosecond laser capsulotomy and manual continuous curvilinear capsulorhexis parameters and their effects on intraocular lens centration. J Refract Surg 2011;27:558–563.
4 Mihaltz K, Knorz MC, Alio JL, Takács AI, Kránitz K, Kovács I, Nagy ZZ: Internal aberration and optical quality after femtosecond laser anterior capsulotomy in cataract surgery. J Refract Surg 2011;27:711–716.
5 Ecsedy M, Mihaltz K, Kovacs I, Takács A, Filkorn T, Nagy ZZ: Effect of femtosecond laser cataract surgery on the macula. J Refract Surg 2011;27:717–722.
6 Takács AI, Kovács I, Miháltz K, Filkorn T, Knorz MC, Nagy ZZ: The effect of femtolaser cataract surgery on the cornea. J Refract Surg, in press.
7 Roberts T, Sutton G, Lawless M, Jindal-Bali S: Capsular blockage syndrome associated with femtosecond laser-assisted cataract surgery. J Cataract Refract Surg 2011;37:2068–2070.

Zoltan Z. Nagy
Department of Ophthalmology, Semmelweis University
Maria u. 39
HU–1085 Budapest (Hungary)
E-Mail zoltan.nagy100@gmail.com

Güell JL (ed): Cataract. ESASO Course Series. Basel, Karger, 2013, vol 3, pp 62–79
DOI: 10.1159/000350909

Laser-Assisted Cataract Surgery with LenSx

Lucio Buratto

Centro Ambrosiano Oftalmico, Milan, Italy

Abstract

To date, innovation and evolution of cataract surgery have included improving the technology of phacoemulsification systems, the design, materials and types of intraocular lenses to allow patients to see at all distances with minimal visual aberrations, and the viscoelastic substances to satisfy the needs of surgeons. Now, the femtosecond laser has marked the beginning of a new age, in which cataract surgery is approached differently with the first part of the surgery performed by the laser which can be programmed and executed without blades in an extraordinarily precise and reproducible manner; this can help to remove an important variable – the human factor, linked to the surgeon's skill and experience, which are subjective factors.

Routine cataract surgery has now become refractive surgery – patients have grown to expect emmetropia and to be primarily spectacle independent. And if that was not enough, they rightly expect good quality of vision, so there is increased pressure on eye surgeons to provide high-quality vision. The main objective of surgery is still to restore the best visual acuity possible considering the conditions of the eye, but there are also increased expectations of good vision without detectable aberrations.

To achieve this aim, what is required is the most 'accurate' surgery possible, reducing or correcting preexisting refractive errors, preventing the induction of astigmatism, preserving the ability to focus at near in many cases and, in general, ensuring high-quality vision, avoiding alterations or damage to the cornea, retina and vitreous.

Femtosecond laser surgery is precise, safe, reliable, accurate and reproducible. These features can improve the surgical outcome, making this a bright future for cataract surgery (table 1).

The term 'femtosecond' comes from the duration of each laser impulse, which lasts only a tiny fraction of a second. The diameter of each laser spot is less than 2 μm and the light's wavelength is in the infrared spectrum (1,053 nm).

In theory, the laser beam (IR wavelength) can be focused on any intraocular tissue with the energy raised to a threshold that causes what is called optical breakdown at the focal point. The high energy released in a very short time interval creates plasma, which is followed by cavitation bubbles and a wave. To cut or separate tissues, the distance between one spot and the next must be appropriate, the succession between one spot and the next must be short, and the energy must be released in precise patterns that can be programmed by the operating surgeon. Considering the diameters involved, numerous laser emissions are required.

Table 1. Advantages and limitations of the femtosecond laser

Advantages
Offer a precise, circular capsulotomy of the desidered size and site
Can reduce the ultrasound energy required during phacoemulsification
Can reduce the amount of fluid circulating in the eye
Can reduce instrument movements in the eye
Can reduce the time of intraocular surgery (but not the overall duration of the operation)
Surgeons can perform surgery without knives/blades or other cutting instruments, which is psychologically very
  important for patients
Corneal incisions are created more accurately and with the same characteristics (reproducibility)

Limitations
The current limitation is the high price; however, at the time of writing, femto-technology has already become
  common practice in over 300 international surgery centers of excellence

---

After paying homage to the pioneering work of Kelman, the father of phacoemulsification (which over 100 million people in the world benefitted from), a second revolution takes place in the field of cataract surgery, the age of femtolaser is beginning.

The energy provided by this laser has, for many years, allowed refractive surgeons to create corneal incisions and flaps with accuracy, precision and reproducibility using robotic tools for most of the surgery and keeping side effects to a minimum. Cataract surgeons expect this laser to provide the same level of precise cutting in many steps of the cataract procedure.

To date, innovation and evolution of cataract surgery have included improving the technology of phacoemulsification systems (with the aim of improving fluidics and reducing trauma to eye tissue), the design, materials and types of intraocular lenses to allow patients to see at all distances with minimal visual aberrations, and the viscoelastic substances (VES) to satisfy the needs of surgeons. Yet, until now no one thought of removing the last variable – the human factor, linked to the surgeon's skill and experience, which are subjective factors.

The femtosecond laser has marked the beginning of a new age, in which cataract surgery is approached differently with the first part of the surgery performed by the laser which can be programmed and executed without blades, in an extraordinarily precise and reproducible manner. This device creates clear corneal incisions, corneal relaxing incisions for the correction of astigmatism (if necessary), anterior capsulotomy, and nuclear fragmentation.

All these procedures are computer programmed and are reproducible every time the laser is used with the same characteristics.

Corneal Incisions

Corneal incisions (corneal tunnel and paracentesis) are performed with great accuracy by programming the desired incisional architecture. The site of incision is chosen according to preoperative topographic values and surgeon preference and intraoperative pachymetry values provided by the optical coherent light tomography (OCT). The surgeon chooses the shape and size of the tunnel, with two or three planes, with different inclination, depth, width, shape and length. The surgeon also chooses the site – temporal, superior or elsewhere – with the aid of the integrated OCT.

The corneal tunnel – a multiplanar incision on two or three levels – during and after the sur-

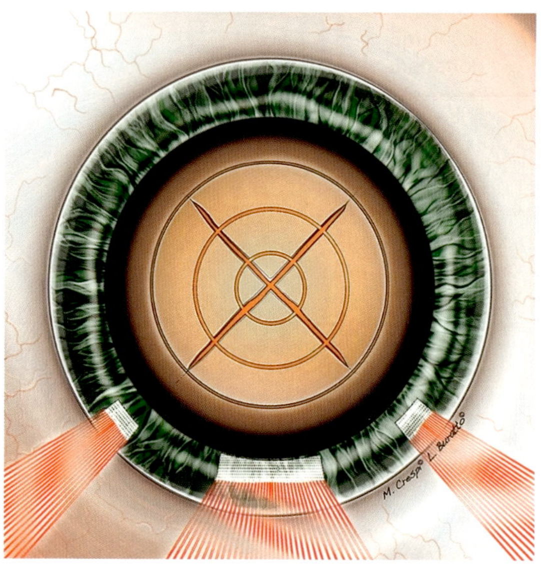

Fig. 1. Laser executes the main incision first and the second ones after.

pending on the amount of astigmatism, corneal thickness, age and pupil diameter. It is therefore easier to perform incisions that are exactly on the axis of astigmatism, perfectly symmetrical (in the case of symmetrical astigmatism or, if this is not the case, asymmetrical), and at the same distance from the pupil. This result is difficult to achieve with manual incisions.

Another important unique feature of femtosecond laser keratotomy is that incisions may be just intrastromal, i.e. without cuts in the epithelium and Bowman's membrane. This spares the patient the symptoms typically associated with corneal wounds and allows the surgeon to decide whether the incisions need to be opened or not (to increase the reduction of astigmatism) after surgery.

gery has excellent flap apposition and is easy to close. This is associated with a lower risk of complications (such as loss of fluid from the wound and the entry of external secretions into the anterior chamber), which should reduce the risk of endophthalmitis (fig. 1).

Various parameters of paracentesis (one or two) can be programmed, such as shape, distance from the main incision, size (width and length) and, naturally, the site(s).

When performing corneal relaxing incisions, moderate astigmatic errors can be corrected by using the laser to perform keratotomy procedures in exactly the desired location, of exactly the desired depth and angle length, which cannot be achieved in keratotomies performed manually with steel or diamond knives.

The unique and special feature of relaxing incisions performed with laser technology is that surgeons can tailor the procedure to each patient, performing different treatment patterns based on the diameter of the optic zone, the length and depth of the incision and the incision angle, de-

Capsulotomy

Capsulotomy is often a challenging procedure for inexperienced surgeons and can be difficult for experienced surgeons as well. With the femtosecond laser, a few seconds is all it takes to perform a perfectly circular capsulotomy of the desired size at the desired site (capsulotomies of different shapes can also be performed by programming the laser) (fig. 2). These aspects are currently important for the insertion of premium IOLs whose performance depends in part on the shape and site of the anterior capsulotomy in order to avoid decentration caused by asymmetric vector forces or contraction of the capsular bag because of irregular shape.

Nuclear Fragmentation

The fragmentation pattern must be set by the surgeon according to the degree of nuclear density and surgical preferences. The femtolaser's software can be programmed to make linear and/ or circular cuts in the crystalline lens, similar to

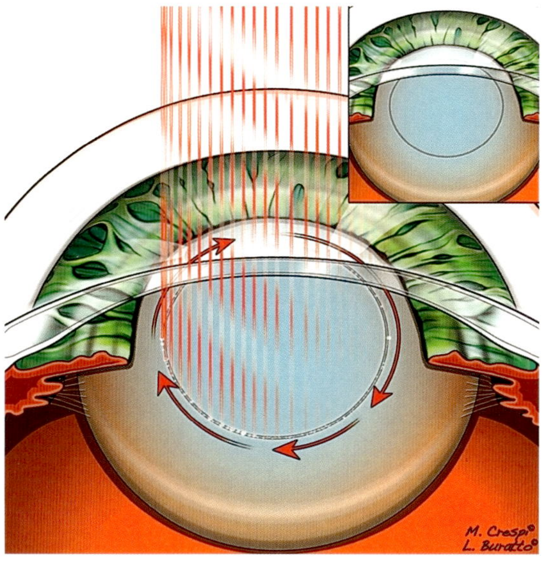

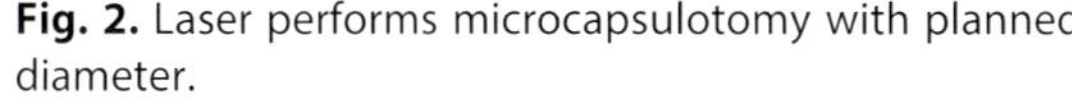

Fig. 2. Laser performs microcapsulotomy with planned diameter.

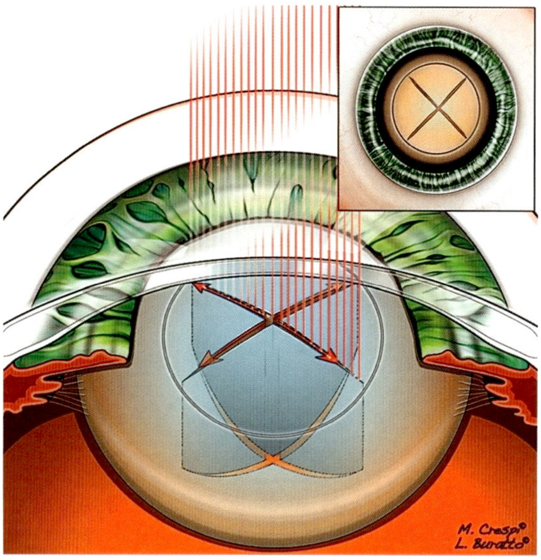

Fig. 3. Laser cuts the nucleus in two, four or more parts.

the latitude and longitude lines on a globe (fig. 3). In the second part of the operation, the lens material can be removed with a phacoemulsification device using only vacuum (if the nucleus is soft) or very low amounts of energy (if the nucleus is moderately hard). Ultrasound-induced trauma on the eye tissue (zonules in particular) and endothelial cell loss are minimized.

Pretreating the nucleus with laser makes the removal of cataracts (even dense ones) easier and quicker (with reduced trauma) because the precise, linear cuts allow cleavage planes to propagate inside the crystalline lens, whereas circular ablations cut the central core of the nucleus, making it softer and easier to remove. Femtolasers allow surgeons to use reduced ultrasound energy for all nuclei and, most importantly, limit the amount of energy required for dense ones. Another consequence is the reduced use of BSS.

A number of laser platforms, with differing features, are currently commercially available. The four companies that have developed the femtosecond lasers are: (1) LenSx Laser Inc. (Al-

iso Viejo, Calif., USA); (2) LensAR Inc. (Winter Park, Fla., USA); (3) OptiMedica Corporation (Santa Ana, Calif., USA); and (4) TPV Technolas (Munich, Germany).

LenSx (Alcon) and Catalys (Optimedica) use 3-D OCT to guide the laser in the eye and to create self-sealing corneal incisions.

LenSx at the beginning used a rigid, curvilinear patient interface (PI). By late 2013, a new PI was released using a disposable soft contact lens, which provides improved docking, improved quality of the capsulotomy, and minimal increase in IOP.

Catalys uses a liquid interface that provides the best contact with the eye without requiring a significant increase in ocular pressure.

Topcon's LensAR, originally designed to correct presbyopia, uses a Scheimpflug camera-based biometric system and develops a cubic pattern of laser impulses that divide the crystalline lens into small, die-shaped parts.

Victus (by Technolas) has a simple docking technique, and the instrument is guided by real-

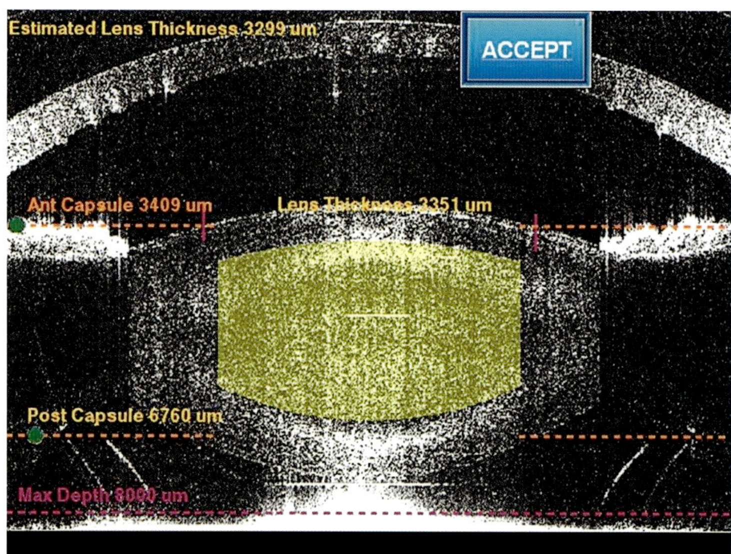

Fig. 4. View of laser OCT for intra-ocular structure measures.

time OCT during the entire laser procedure, ensuring accurate measurement of intraocular elements (the crystalline lens in particular), as well as providing an excellent image of the anterior and posterior capsule of the crystalline lens. Surgeons who wish to perform keratotomy procedures using Victus must perform a second docking with a different PI than that used for the laser fragmentation of the crystalline lens.

Optical Coherent Light Tomography

LenSx has a high-resolution OCT system. This method – first developed for ophthalmology – has been used in diagnostics of the anterior and posterior segments of the eye for a number of years, but this is the first time it has been used on a 'surgical' instrument.

OCT is a noninvasive imaging technique that yields excellent results in medical imaging and in measuring the components of the human eye. OCT images are acquired by transmitting energy waves into the tissue and measuring the echo of the reflected waves. The 'streaked' appearance of images of homogeneous tissue such as the cornea are an effect of the granularity caused by the coherent light used in OCT.

OCT generates transverse images of the components of the eye and provides a direct, high-resolution image, without contact with the eye, making this a non-invasive technique. The axial resolution of the image is 10 μm at a 1,310-nm wavelength. The size of the acquisition slice is about 10 mm.

OCT imaging does not just provide a qualitative assessment of the various eye tissues – it can supply quantitative information, since it can be used to measure the thickness, diameter and anomalies of the eye profile and the homogeneity of tissue. This is useful in the OCT devices used in femtosecond lasers (fig. 4).

Femtolaser Surgery

There are two distinct steps:
- The laser component, with predocking programming, the application of the suction ring, docking, OCT, post-programming of

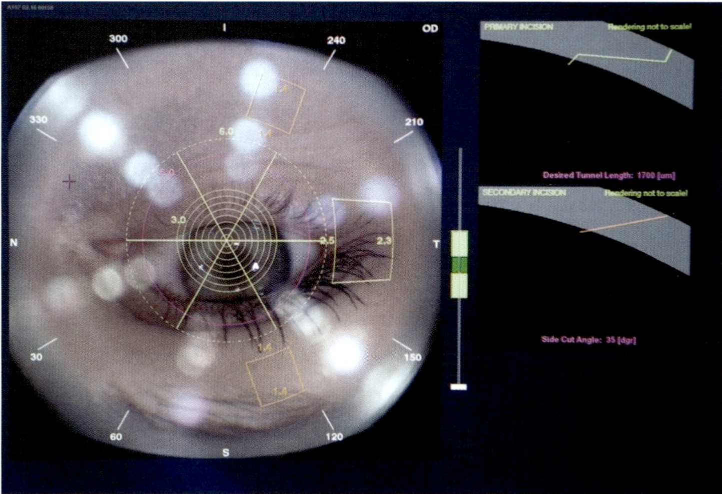

Fig. 5. Programming laser treatment.

the laser treatment and the execution of the laser phase.

– The surgical component, in which the surgeon opens one of the incisions, injects VES, removes the capsule, opens the second and third incisions (if done), performs careful hydrodissection, removes the nucleus, then removes the cortex and implants the IOL.

Laser Phase

Pre-Docking Programming

Before starting the laser procedure on a patient, the surgeon must program what is desired from the laser, e.g. the position, shape, width, architecture and length of the primary incision and the accessory incision(s). The size of the capsulotomy must be programmed.

A pattern must be chosen for nuclear fragmentation (which depends on the density of the nucleus and other parameters). The surgeon must also choose a cylindrical, linear or mixed pattern and appropriate dimensions. The energy of each individual spot, the distance between one shot and the next, the emission frequency and the succession must be established before patient treatment with any of the procedures above. This typically remains fixed (fig. 5).

Laser Treatment of the Patient

The surgeon must apply a few drops of topical anesthetic, insert an adjustable lid speculum and adjust it to obtain a wide palpebral aperture. The patient's head should be on a firm cushion on the stretcher and parallel with the floor, allowing maximal and equal conjunctival exposure. The suction ring is applied so that the integrated OCT device may take accurate measurements and after subsequent programming, direct the laser to the correct depth and placement. Additionally, it prevents eye movement during laser emission, obviously undesirable.

The next step in the procedure is docking, i.e. bringing the laser device in contact with the eye. Docking consists in allowing the cornea and the surrounding conjunctiva to adhere to a special plastic 'cone' called the PI with suction. The PI must allow the OCT device in the instrument to scan the anterior segment, i.e. measure the thickness and the distance between the various eye structures involved in cataract surgery (fig. 6).

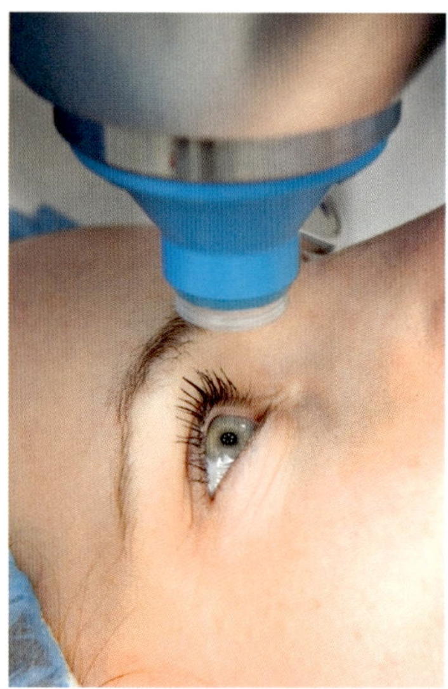

Fig. 6. Docking.

Good docking requires that the applanation is parallel to the anterior and posterior surface of the crystalline lens, so that the laser treatment is performed on planes that are parallel to the structures it needs to interact with.

Using the joystick, the surgeon (or the laser technician) moves the tip of the laser until the PI enters the suction ring and is in contact with the eye. While moving the laser closer to the eye, the surgeon must instruct the patient to fixate into the laser correctly and continuously in order to center it most effectively. An optimal connection between the eye and the PI is very important – other than allowing the OCT device to take accurate measurements, it also leads to faster programming of the laser procedure.

The docking step is the most important part of the laser procedure because if it is performed incorrectly, the measurements taken by the OCT device may be inaccurate, which means that the surgical program may also be inaccurate. It is therefore very important to obtain a stable connection between the eye and the PI and for the PI to be aligned with the laser's optical system. If the laser's optical system is not aligned (if even by the fraction of a millimeter), at least part of the energy will be directed incorrectly, achieving less accurate results and performance or causing complications. If, for example, the applanation made by the PI is not perfectly parallel to the anterior surface of the crystalline lens, the capsulotomy may be incomplete or not perfectly executed. The nucleus may not be sufficiently divided and/or divided into wrong planes (which, extremely rarely, can cause the posterior capsule to break). The corneal incisions may be incorrect, i.e. too anterior or posterior; they could be incomplete or of a different shape from the one desired in the program.

Incorrect docking may also lead to loss of suction during surgery, which terminates the laser procedure and does not allow the surgeon to have the advantages offered by laser treatment. The possible loss of suction during the laser procedure must be immediately noticed. A meniscus or redundant conjunctival tissue appearing on the monitor's screen are clues that can warn about an imminent loss of suction. In these conditions, intraocular procedures can continue in most cases, whereas corneal incision procedures must almost always be stopped and finished surgically. Tight palpebral fissures, pediatric age and flat corneas have been identified as risk factors in loss of suction.

The incidence of loss of suction during LASIK femtosecond laser surgery has been reported to be 0.06–0.27%. There are currently no statistical data on the use of femtosecond laser for cataract surgery, but loss of suction is a complication that may occur.

Good docking can be achieved by making sure the patient is in the correct position, avoiding interference from the nose and talking the patient through the procedure, ensuring he/she looks into the laser. A stable bed with elevation that can be adjusted by the surgeon (to obtain the best bed-patient-laser condition) is also useful.

All the above is not, by itself, enough. An adequate palpebral opening, a distended conjunctiva without significant abnormalities, a conjunctival sac free from liquid and, cooperation from the patient are required – partly because the docking procedure can be uncomfortable and, on the whole, lasts 2–3 min.

Once docking has been performed correctly, the surgeon (or the laser technician) uses the computer keyboard or mouse to program the various treatment steps, one at a time.

To begin with, he/she must check that the OCT device is centered on the eye, then check that the programmed capsulotomy is perfectly centered or slightly decentered as desired on the pupil. Next, he/she must check the OCT projection of the crystalline lens and establish at what depth the laser emission must start and end (usually 500–600 μm from the posterior and the anterior capsule) and therefore the crystalline lens cut. The ablation pattern is selected prior to docking.

Next, the surgeon (or the laser technician) must examine the anterior capsule and ensure it is on a horizontal plane, as this is important to achieve a complete (360°) capsulotomy. To be on the safe side, the operator must program the computer so that the laser treatment begins under the capsule and ends above it. In this way, the capsule is certain to be cut all the way through.

To perform the capsulotomy, laser emission is started 300–400 μm under the capsule (delta down), in the superficial material of the crystalline lens, and gradually moves upwards in a spiral motion (delta up) until it reaches the capsule. It moves into the anterior chamber for 300 μm – this is very important because the capsule thickness may vary in different areas. Furthermore, the crystalline lens (and therefore the capsule) may not be on a perfectly horizontal plane (the crystalline lens may be tilted due to imperfect docking), and this allows the laser emission to compensate for small abnormalities caused by less than perfect docking.

Naturally, in the post-docking programming phase, the surgeon has centered the capsulotomy site as well as possible, whereas the diameter and shape are programmed in the pre-docking phases. Occasionally, despite accurate docking and precise programming, the capsule is not cut 360°, which may depend on other reasons (described below).

Once the laser surgery is fully programmed, the operator presses the pedal that activates the laser and the surgery proper begins. It usually takes 40–50 s of laser time.

The first step is capsulotomy, which is not actually a capsulorhexis but a 'micro can opener'. It is not a continuous opening (like a tear-open lid) but a series of micropunctures or capsular perforations instead. They are very close to each other and the final result is an extremely precise and perfectly circular (and resistant) capsulotomy. Once the capsulotomy is complete, the laser program continues with the programmed procedure in the nucleus. If programmed, corneal relaxing incisions for the correction of astigmatism are performed next, followed by the creation of the main and accessory incisions. The laser procedure is then finished.

Surgery Phase

The patient is moved under the operating microscope and surgery is performed. The surgeon should use the best magnification and light of the microscope to check if the capsulotomy is complete – the surgical procedure is different if there are micro-connections or extensive areas of uncut capsule.

Opening the Incisions
To begin with, using a blunt spatula, the surgeon opens one of the accessory incisions and immediately injects a VES (possibly viscoadhesive, such as Discovisc Alcon, Fort Worth, Texas) in order to avoid shallowing or flattening of the anterior chamber and, possibly, the rupture of the anterior capsule, should there be a point of lower resistance.

Next, the other accessory incision may be opened (if created), then the main incision.

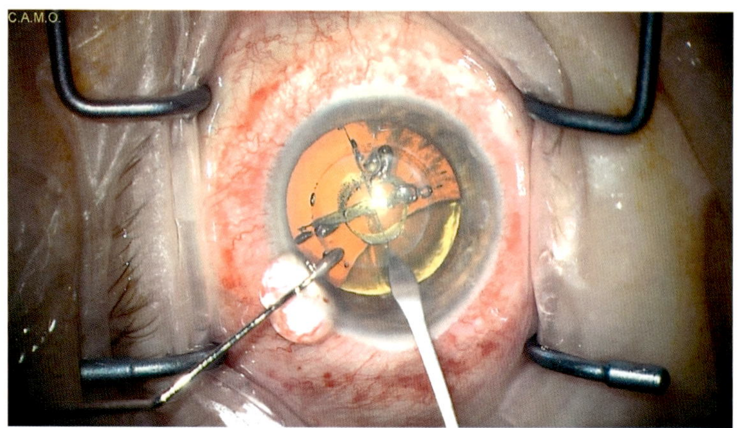

Fig. 7. Opening of the main and secondary incision with a blunt spatula.

Blunt spatulas are used to open the incisions because the opening procedure is actually a dissection of the tissue on which the laser has worked, similar to creation of a flap in the LASIK procedure. It should be noted that the eye is considered closed until the surgeon opens the incisions with the spatula. This means the laser procedure can be performed in a different operating room or even building that is not where surgery is performed. Some time may lapse between the laser procedure and the surgery, even if it is preferable that surgery follows immediately in order to avoid pupil constriction due to the release of energy in the eye (fig. 7).

Removal of the Anterior Capsule
At this point, the anterior capsule may be removed. It is essential that the surgeon confirms that the capsule has been completely cut (360°) or if micro- or macroscopic connections have remained. This information is crucial in determining how to proceed.

The anterior capsule is not always visible because the anterior chamber is often turbid (trypan blue can be very useful in this situation).

Turbidity is essentially caused by two factors. The first factor is the stirring up of cortical material just under the anterior capsule caused by the laser beginning the ablation procedure about 300 μm under the capsule. This reduces the red reflex and, in any case, may not allow the capsule to be viewed clearly.

The second factor is the presence of gas in the nucleus and, in general, under the anterior capsule. The gas is a result of the ablation – the tissue disintegrated by the laser is transformed into gas (plasma) that is trapped in the crystalline lens material and may hinder visualization of the red reflex (and therefore visibility for the surgeon). This occurs mainly in the observation/removal of the anterior capsule as well as during hydrodissection.

The surgeon proceeds differently depending on whether the capsule is perfectly cut (360°) or tissue connections remain.

If the capsule is completely cut (360°), the surgeon can choose between removing the cleaved capsule with forceps or using the aspiration function of the US tip (fig. 8).

Assuming the surgeon removes the capsule with forceps, he/she can follow the traditional phacoemulsification procedure to perform hydrodissection. If this is done, it must be performed cautiously because the capsular bag contains bubbles, which increases its tension and makes it more likely to rupture.

Before carrying out hydrodissection, the surgeon may decide to use phacoemulsification to remove the superficial layer of lens material in order

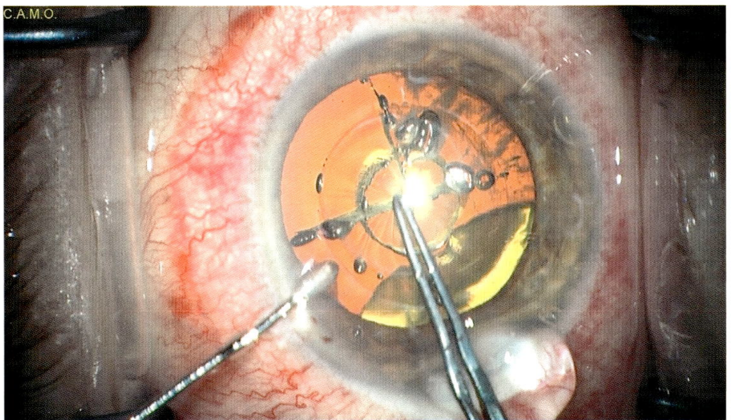

Fig. 8. Removal of the cut anterior capsule.

to obtain better results, aiming at achieving three objectives: (1) To remove part of the anterior cortical material that became loose during the laser emission and during the removal of the anterior capsule. This step improves visibility in the anterior segment and especially of the contents of the capsular bag. (2) To decompress the capsular bag because, by removing some of the lens material, part of the gas that formed in the nucleus can be released and enter the anterior chamber, improving visibility of the nucleus and better see the progression of the hydrodissection BSS wave (that will take place later). (3) To clearly visualize the linear cuts made by the laser (if this was the chosen pattern) and decide to divide the nucleus into two parts with a prechopper, to make the next steps of the procedure easier and to release more plasma bubbles from the lens material (fig. 9). Having done this, visibility in the anterior segment has improved and the red reflex is better.

The surgeon can decide to remove the anterior capsule using the aspiration of the US tip and continue with the phacoaspiration or phacofragmentation of the nucleus. However, the surgeon must be quite sure that the nucleus is soft enough to be easily aspirated even without hydrodissection. Alternatively, the surgeon must have good bimanual dexterity and be able to perform hydrodissection with the non-dominant hand and use the phaco-handpiece with the dominant hand.

In the case of incomplete capsulotomy, the surgeon must complete the capsulotomy using capsulorhexis forceps. Great caution is required in this step in order to avoid a residual tissue connection transforming into capsulorhexis escape. This is the most challenging and difficult step the surgeon has to manage after initial treatment with the femtosecond laser for cataract surgery. Poor visibility of the capsule and the presence of a plasma bubble-filled capsular bag can make completing the capsulotomy very difficult.

The use of trypan blue and injection of an appropriate viscoadhesive substance (Discovisc) can greatly help the surgeon.

After removing the anterior capsule (and eventually some of the anterior lens material), the surgeon may elect to proceed with careful hydrodissection, carefully observing the progression of the BSS wave that separates the posterior capsule from the posterior epinuclear material (fig. 10).

Hydrodissection
This step must be performed with caution and without injecting too much BSS in the capsular bag, which may already be expanded by the presence of the bubbles.

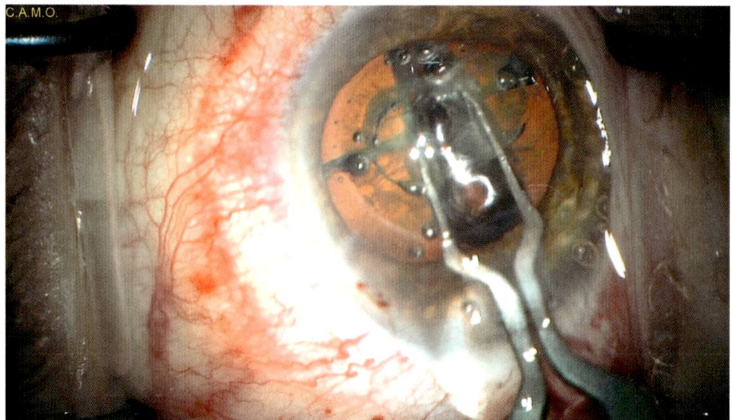

Fig. 9. Nucleus prechopping.

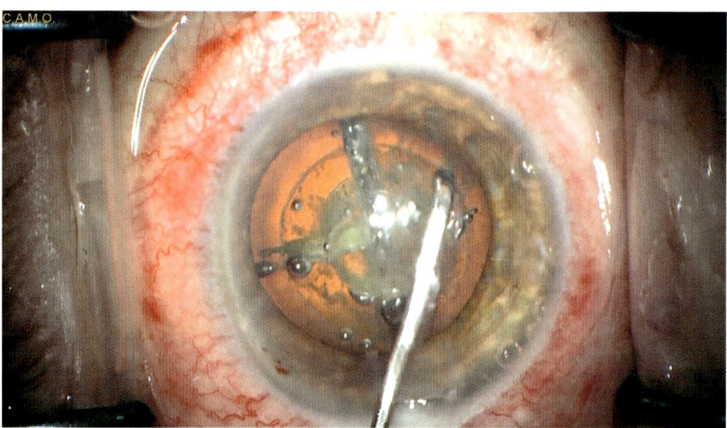

Fig. 10. Careful hydrodissection.

At the end of hydrodissection, rotation of the nucleus in the capsular bag (to be certain it is not connected to the bag any more) should be performed.

Phacoemulsification

At this point, phacoemulsification may begin. The technique to be used depends on the density of the nucleus and, in the case of femtolaser-treated nuclei, on the nuclear dissection pattern used. However, it is important to bear in mind that the cuts in the crystalline lens material are not complete and the deeper layer remains uncut. The surgeon must be able to deal with a nucleus that is divided only centrally and has a 'posterior bowl' that is not cut because of its proximity to the posterior capsule. In this case – especially if the nucleus is soft or not very dense – it is advisable to proceed with flipping the epinucleus after removing the inner, harder nucleus. Usually, if the nucleus is of the appropriate consistency, a prechopper can be used to divide the nucleus and the deeper layer that has not been cut by the laser, or this may be accomplished using the phaco-tip and the second instrument, spatula or chopper (fig. 11).

Most femto-surgeons prefer to use a laser with a cylindrical pattern on nuclei considered

Buratto

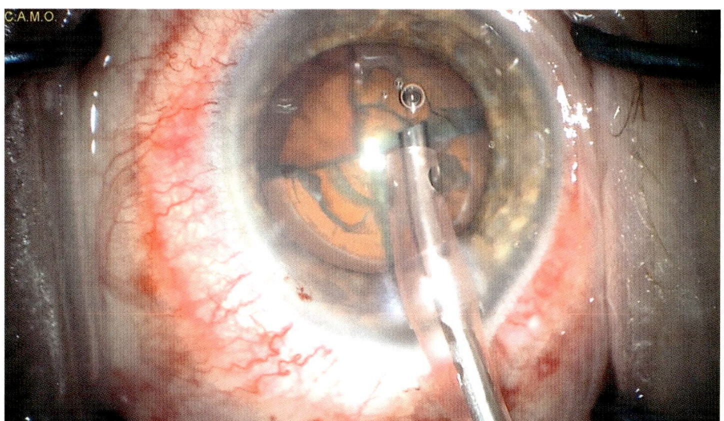

Fig. 11. Quadrant phacoemulsification.

soft or not very hard before surgery. The cylindrical pattern has the advantage of further softening an already soft nucleus, which can then be removed simply using the irrigation/aspiration handpiece or the US handpiece without ultrasound.

To cut hard nuclei, femto-surgeons mostly use a laser pattern that divides the nucleus into 2, 4, 6 or 8 parts.

Surgeons must be aware that laser ablation does not 'cut' and that tissue connections remain. A chopper is therefore required to separate the sectors completely. Alternatively, a prechopper can be used before phacoemulsification.

The nucleus division pattern can also be mixed, i.e. there may be one or more cylinders combined with one or more linear divisions. When dealing with hard or semi-hard nuclei, it is very useful to perform a 3-mm cylindrical cut and two to three linear cross-incisions, which allow the surgeon to remove the four central parts of the nucleus first. After dividing the nucleus into 4 parts with a prechopper or a chopper, the four sections can be removed very easily using the 'quadrant removal' parameters of Infiniti (Alcon) with the Ozil system (fig. 11).

If the nucleus was cut into 4 or 6 sectors, the anterior epinucleus must be removed first. The surgeon may then use a chopper to fully divide the sectors and remove them using a standard technique.

The I/A Tip
After phacoemulsification, the cortex must be removed (fig. 12). Many femto-surgeons have noted that more cortex remains, and it is more adherent to the anterior and posterior capsule.

This is probably secondary to the more cautious hydrodissection performed after femtofragmentation of the nucleus, as well as the fact that the anterior cortical material is cleanly cut during the capsulotomy, without the tags typically left after manual capsulorhexis. It could also be caused by the gas bubbles released in the capsular bag that make the cortex adhere to the capsule more strongly.

The cortex can be removed with the I/A coaxial tip or with the Buratto bimanual technique. In femtolaser surgery, the latter procedure has many advantages, as it allows the chamber to be deep during the entire procedure and, most importantly, to access every part of the capsular bag without inducing excessive pressure or traction on the incisions.

New Instruments
Using a femtosecond laser leads to changes in surgery technique and, therefore, to the use of new instruments. A small, flat spatula with a blunt tip is required to open the corneal incisions. A pre-

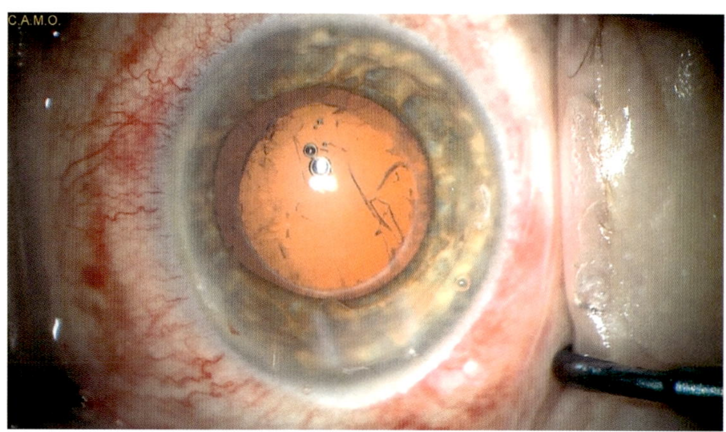
Fig. 12. Residual cortex after phacoemulsification.

chopper with a new design is needed to fully divide the nucleus after laser phacofragmentation. Special forceps – suitable for gripping the anterior capsule and detaching residual capsular connections – are necessary.

Contraindications to Femtolaser Surgery
Possible indications and contraindications to the operation are essentially associated with the following factors: (1) characteristics of the conjunctiva; (2) exposure of the eye; (3) general conditions such as patient cooperation/anxiety; (4) transparency of the cornea; (5) diameter of the pupil; and (6) depth of the anterior chamber.

Conjunctiva
Anything that hinders correct docking is a contraindication to laser treatment. A post-glaucoma surgery bleb, conjunctival or palpebral pathologies that limit palpebral opening, even loose conjunctiva can make correct docking impossible, which means no laser surgery can be performed.

It is important to bear in mind that there are considerable differences between docking for LASIK and docking for cataract surgery. The former only needs contact with the cornea, includes the ablation of the superficial layers of the cornea, is performed quickly, requires low energy, raises intraocular pressure quite a lot, and the

surface of contact with the cornea is flat. Docking for cataract surgery requires the suction ring to adhere to the conjunctiva, OCT procedures must be performed, ablation mainly involves intraocular tissue, laser times are longer, the contact surface is curved to follow the curvature of the cornea better and induces less increase in intraocular pressure.

Exposure of the Eye
Very deep-set eyes, an excessively prominent nose, reduced palpebral opening, a cornea that is too curved or too flat can make docking ineffective and therefore laser-assisted surgery cannot be performed.

General Conditions
Lack of cooperation from patients for health reasons (Alzheimer's, paralysis, muscular deficit and systemic pathologies) or excess anxiety can be contraindications to surgery. Nystagmus may be a contraindication only if eye movement is excessive.

Transparency of the Cornea
To achieve its goal, the laser beam must release its energy into the crystalline lens without interference. Any corneal opacity or nebula can reduce or block the passage of laser beams. This mainly

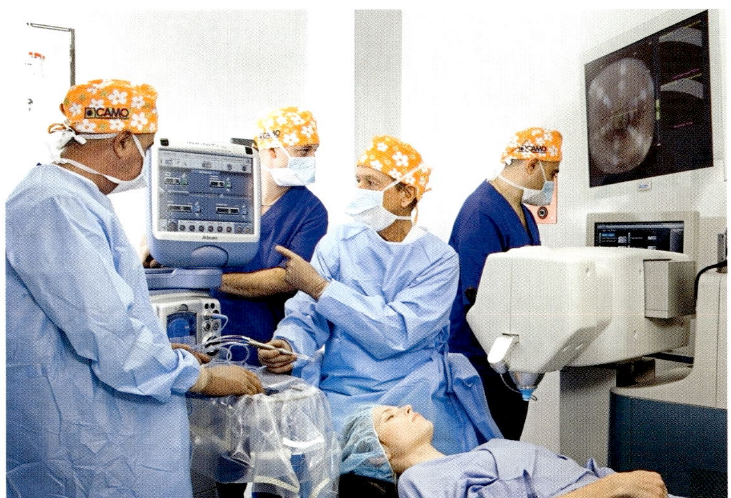

Fig. 13. Staff, laser and phaco-emulsification equipment ready for surgery.

affects the capsulotomy that may be incomplete. The same applies to the action on the lens material and/or corneal tissue, even if this is less important in the general context of the operation.

Likewise, corneal edema (caused by some pathologies of the cornea) can limit or block the transmission of the laser.

Diameter of the Pupil

In most cases, surgeons desire a capsulotomy centered on the pupil, with a diameter between 4.5 and 5.5 mm. Laser emission should also be at least 1 mm from the edge of the pupil, so that iris pigment does not interfere with the passage of the laser energy (and also because excessive proximity stimulates miosis of the pupil). Patients with a small pupil, pupils with synechiae or decentered pupils may not be suitable for laser surgery.

Depth of the Anterior Chamber

Increased distance between the cornea and the anterior capsule of the lens does not affect laser surgery, but a shallow chamber could do so because the laser emission for capsulotomy may be too close to the endothelium and damage this important layer of cells (fig. 13).

Side Effects and Complications

As with any new technology, there is a learning curve associated with the use of the femtosecond laser for cataract surgery. This technique – like any other surgical procedure – is not free of side effects and complications, mainly intraoperative. It has been shown that the greater the number of operations performed, the lower the percentage of complications (the decrease is significant). After the first 50 cases (learning curve), complications such as capsulotomy escape or capsular rupture and/or dislocation of lens material into the vitreous decrease dramatically.

To begin with, surgeons must learn to align the eye with the laser's optical system, to interpret the tomography images and to adjust the laser's parameters correctly. If these steps are not performed properly, they can lead to complications and side effects that even experienced surgeons may not be well equipped to manage.

Listed below are the main problems that still need improvement:

Difficulties Making the Incisions

It is sometimes difficult to position the entrance of the tunnel for phacoemulsification correctly during the programming phase. If the entrance ends up in a vascularized area or in any non-transparent area of the cornea, the corneal incision will be incomplete and the surgeon will have to use a knife. The same applies to accessory incisions.

Sometimes, the position of the incision ends up being too anterior in the cornea, which makes intraocular maneuvers challenging. The incision can be too oblique, which hinders the surgeon and can induce mild, irregular astigmatism.

Finally, relaxing incisions for the correction of astigmatism require nomograms that make the results more predictable and reproducible.

Problems Obtaining a Complete Capsulotomy

This can be caused by a number of factors, such as corneal folds induced by docking (which can interfere with the laser beam propagating evenly and uniformly), more or less opaque areas in the cornea, scars left by wounds or ulcers, scars resulting from corneal surgery – all can interfere with optimal transmission of laser energy.

Dishomogeneous capsular density can cause incomplete cut. However, delta up and delta down associated with the correct quantity of energy emitted per shot make this occurrence rare.

Other factors causing incomplete capsulotomy, as mentioned above, are docking with tilting or loss of suction during laser emission.

Palanker and colleagues reported the presence of microgrooves at the edge of the anterior capsulotomy, with the formation of small folds that can make capsular ruptures more likely to develop. For this reason, it is important that the capsulotomy is completed manually with forceps, with the aim of stopping the microincisions of the anterior capsular edge from spreading equatorially and posteriorly.

If loss of suction occurs during laser emission, the femtocapsulotomy will be incomplete. In this case, an experienced surgeon can repeat the docking procedure and program a larger diameter for the capsulotomy.

Presence of Lens Dust in the Anterior Chamber That Reduces Visibility

This problem may arise during removal of the anterior capsule and during hydrodissection. As mentioned above, the emission of the laser spots begins 300–400 μm below the anterior capsule (delta down) and ends about 300 μm above (delta up). Laser emission therefore occurs intensely also on the anterior epinucleus, which causes lens dust to move, and some of it will enter the anterior chamber through the incisions of the anterior capsule, reducing visibility for the surgeon.

Another important element that limits visibility to surgeons is the presence of plasma bubbles in the lens material. The higher the energy released in the lens, the larger the amount of bubbles. Bubbles are also related to the segmentation pattern.

Visibility is also reduced if a cylindrical pattern is used because the cylinders affect the very core of the nucleus and are below the capsulotomy. Furthermore, they are very close to each other and create turbidity.

Partial Constriction of the Pupil

Intraoperative miosis is the result of the emission of laser energy in the anterior chamber and near the pupil margin and may be caused by direct stimulation of the iris or release of prostaglandin. Miosis can make phacoemulsification more difficult and hinder correct positioning of the IOL, especially with toric or special designs. This side effect, which can be a problem for the surgeon, can in part be prevented by adding a drop of 10% phenylephrine at the end of the laser procedure and before the actual surgery. To prevent laser-induced miosis, the use of a 1% atropine solution before surgery and the use of preservative-free adrenalin in the irrigation bottle during surgery can help. The time between the laser procedure and surgery should be as short as possible.

The Need to Perform Hydrodissection Very
Delicately
The capsular bag has already been distended by the
bubbles released during laser ablation, so delicate
hydrodissection is necessary to prevent the volume
of the capsular bag from expanding (which could
ultimately cause the bag to rupture). Inadequate
hydrodissection is associated with a number of
small problems that make the operation more
complex.

To begin with, the epinucleus and the cortex
adhere more strongly, so more traction and time
are required to remove them. This may also be
caused by the fact that the gas bubbles released
when the nuclear incisions are created make the
cortex adhere more strongly to the residual anterior and equatorial posterior capsule.

Furthermore, more fragments of the lens remain on the posterior capsule, which require scra-
ping/cleaning procedures of the posterior capsule
that take longer than those with traditional hydrodissection after capsulorhexis with forceps or
a cystotome.

In any case, the removal of the cortex is easier
to perform with the Buratto bimanual technique
because it is easier to access the capsular bag (360°).

Incomplete Fragmentation of the Nucleus
The effect of the laser may not be sufficient to segment very dense nuclei, so the ablation may not
create defined grooves that can be transformed
into cuts using a prechopper, chopper or other
tools for nuclear fragmentation.

In most cases, the surgeon must be able to
manage a nucleus where only the surface is fragmented, and there is a 'posterior bowl' of nucleus
that was not fragmented because of proximity to
the posterior capsule. If the cataract is not hard,
flipping the nucleus or sculpting to achieve complete fragmentation is recommended.

The Formation of Large Gas Bubbles
Some appear immediately in the anterior chamber, along the edges of the capsulotomy. Other

gas bubbles form inside the lens nucleus and can
cause iatrogenic damage. The gas generated during the laser procedure increases the intracapsu-
lar volume and rarely – in inappropriately managed cases – the posterior capsule may break and
the lens may be dislocated into the vitreous humor. This is partly caused by an increase in intra-
capsular pressure, but primarily by incorrect hydrodissection that can further increase intracap-
sular pressure.

Predisposing factors include: posterior polar
cataracts, mature cataracts, long axial length and
rapid, excessive hydrodissection.

To avoid this complication, surgeons should:
-   avoid filling the anterior chamber completely
    with viscoelastic material before removing
    the anterior capsule;
-   lift the edge of the anterior capsule during
    hydrodissection;
-   inject the fluid for hydrodissection slowly
    using the expansion of the visible wave as a
    reference point;
-   decompress the anterior chamber before and
    during hydrodissection by applying pressure
    on the posterior lip of the corneal incision;
-   there is no doubt that the most effective
    method is using a prechopper or a chopper
    (or even a cannula) to fragment the nucleus
    of the lens, in order to release the gas and/or
    liquid, and performing hydrodissection only
    after the release has occurred.

Posterior Capsular Rupture and Nucleus
Dislocations
This is mainly caused by radial tears in the anterior capsule extending posteriorly. It is crucial
that any microincisions at the edge of the capsulotomy are anticipated and managed carefully.
The microincisions are caused by the incomplete
incision of the capsule by the laser or because the
surgeon is unable to see capsular connections remaining after the laser treatment or by other factors (tilting of the lens, corneal opacity and capsular thickening).

Inability to Perform Infiltration Anesthesia
Performing any kind of infiltration anesthesia before the laser treatment is not suitable because it would hinder the docking process. Infiltration anesthesia, if needed, can be performed after laser treatment and before phacoemulsification.

It can be said that the femtosecond laser is the road to follow to further improve cataract surgery – the next steps will be the use of laser in other steps of the procedure, the liquefaction of the crystalline lens and new, increasingly customized IOLs.

As the Russian philosopher and revolutionary Mikhail Bakunin said, 'By striving to do the impossible, man has always achieved what is possible. Those who have cautiously done no more than they believed possible have never taken a single step forward.'

Suggested Reading

1 Miyake K, Ota I, Ichihashi S, Miyake S, Tanaka Y, Terasaki H: New classification of capsular block syndrome. J Cataract Refract Surg 1998;24:1230–1234.
2 Luna JD, Artal MN, Reviglio VE, Pelizzari M, Diaz H, Juarez CP: Vitreoretinal alterations following laser in situ keratomileusis: clinical and experimental studies. Graefes Arch Clin Exp Ophthalmol 2001;239:416–423.
3 Smith RJ, Yadarola MB, Pelizzari MF, Luna JD, Juarez CP, Reviglio VE: Complete bilateral vitreous detachment after LASIK retreatment. J Cataract Refract Surg 2004;30:1382–1384.
4 Mirshahi A, Kohnen T: Effect of microkeratome suction during LASIK on ocular structures. Ophthalmology 2005;112:645–649.
5 Misra A, Burton RL: Incidence of intraoperative complications during phacoemulsification in vitrectomized and nonvitrectomized eyes: prospective study. J Cataract Refract Surg 2005;31:1011–1014.
6 Marques FF, Marques DM, Osher RH, Osher JM: Fate of anterior capsule tears during cataract surgery. J Cataract Refract Surg 2006;32:1638–1642.
7 Binder PS: One thousand consecutive IntraLase laser in situ keratomileusis flaps. J Cataract Refract Surg 2006;32:962–969.
8 Davis RM, Evangelista JA: Ocular structure changes during vacuum by the Hansatome microkeratome suction ring. J Refract Surg 2007;23:563–566.
9 Zaidi FH, Corbett MC, Burton BJ, Bloom PA: Raising the benchmark for the 21st century – the 1000 cataract operations audit and survey: outcomes, consultant-supervised training and sourcing NHS choice. Br J Ophthalmol 2007;91:731–736.
10 Koplin RS, Anderson JE, Seedor JA, Ritterband DC: In situ nuclear disassembly: efficient phacoemulsification without nuclear rotation using lateral sweep sculpting and in situ cracking techniques. J Cataract Refract Surg 2009;35:1487–1491.
11 Haft P, Yoo SH, Kymionis GD, Ide T, O'Brien TP, Culbertson WW: Complications of LASIK flaps made by the IntraLase 15- and 30-kHz femtosecond lasers. J Refract Surg 2009;25:979–984.
12 Jaycock P, Johnston RL, Taylor H, Adams M, Tole DM, Galloway P, Canning C, Sparrow JM: The Cataract National Dataset electronic multi-centre audit of 55,567 operations: updating benchmark standards of care in the United Kingdom and internationally. Eye (Lond) 2009;23:38–49.
13 Nagy Z: Intraocular femtosecond laser applications in cataract surgery: precise laser incisions may enable surgeons to deliver more reproducible outcomes. Cataract Refract Surg Today 2009;9:29–30.
14 Nagy Z, Takacs A, Filkorn T, Sarayba M: Initial clinical evaluation of an intraocular femtosecond laser in cataract surgery. J Refract Surg 2009;25:1053–1060.
15 Conway ML, Wevill M, Benavente-Perez A, Hosking SL: Ocular blood-flow hemodynamics before and after application of a laser in situ keratomileusis ring. J Cataract Refract Surg 2010;36:268–272.
16 Palanker DV, Blumenkranz MS, Andersen D, Wiltberger M, Marcellino G, Gooding P, Angeley D, Schuele G, Woodley B, Simoneau M, Friedman NJ, Seibel B, Batlle J, Feliz R, Talamo J, Culbertson W: Femtosecond laser-assisted cataract surgery with integrated optical coherence tomography. Sci Transl Med 2010;2:58ra85.
17 Slade SG, Culbertson WW, Kreuger RR: Femtosecond lasers for refractive cataract surgery. Cataract Refract Surg Today 2010;10:67–69.
18 Dick H: Femtosecond laser in ophthalmology – a short overview of current applications. Med Laser Appl 2010;25:258–261.
19 Clark A, Morlet N, Ng JQ, Preen DB, Semmens JB: Whole population trends in complications of cataract surgery over 22 years in Western Australia. Ophthalmology 2011;118:1055–1061.
20 Miháltz K, Knorz MC, Alió JL, Takács AI, Kránitz K, Kovács I, Nagy ZZ: Internal aberrations and optical quality after femtosecond laser anterior capsulotomy in cataract surgery. J Refract Surg 2011;27:711–716.
21 Friedman NJ, Palanker DV, Schuele G, Andersen D, Marcellino G, Seibel BS, Batlle J, Feliz R, Talamo JH, Blumenkranz MS, Culbertson WW: Femtosecond laser capsulotomy. J Cataract Refract Surg 2011;37:1189–1198.
22 Ecsedy M, Mihaltz K, Kovacs I, Takács A, Filkorn T, Nagy ZZ: Effect of femtosecond laser cataract surgery on the macula. J Refract Surg 2011;27:717–722.

23 Auffarth G: Preliminary clinical results of the femto-cataract procedure using the VICTUS™ femtosecond laser platform; white paper, September 2011.

24 Bali SJ, Hodge C, Lawless M, Roberts TV, Sutton G: Early experience with the femtosecond laser for cataract surgery. Ophthalmology 2012;119:891–899.

25 Roberts TV, Lawless M, Chan CC, Jacobs M, Ng D, Bali SJ, Hodge C, Sutton G: Femtosecond laser cataract surgery: technology and clinical practice. Clin Experiment Ophthalmol 2013;41:180–186.

26 Álvarez-Rementeria L: Surgical induced astigmatism in femtosecond laser assisted cataract surgery. J Emetropia 2012;3:61–65.

27 Hodge C: Femtosecond cataract surgery: a review of current literature and the experience from an initial installation. Saudi J Ophthalmol 2012;26:73–78.

28 Packer M: LENSAR laser system applications in refractive cataract surgery. S Cataract Refract Surg Today 2012: 3–6.

Lucio Buratto
Centro Ambrosiano Oftalmico
Piazza della Repubblica 21
IT–20124 Milan (Italy)
E-Mail iol.lasik@buratto.com

Güell JL (ed): Cataract. ESASO Course Series. Basel, Karger, 2013, vol 3, pp 80–99
DOI: 10.1159/000350911

Phakic Intraocular Lenses

François Malecaze · Marie Porterie · Myriam Cassagne

Department of Ophthalmology, Purpan Hospital, Toulouse, France

Abstract

Phakic intraocular lenses (pIOLs) implantation concerns high ametropia. Initially developed for high myopia correction, the treatment fields were expanded to astigmatism and hyperopia corrections. Three basic types of pIOLs allow these corrections: anterior chamber IOLs, iris-fixated IOLs and posterior chamber IOLs. Each one has its own complications: the main side effect of anterior or iris-fixated IOLs is the corneal endothelial cells loss, whereas the principal risk of posterior chamber IOLs is anterior subcapsular cataract formation. The risk of glaucoma development exists with all pIOLs. Thus, pIOLs implantation should be proposed cautiously to patients and offered to those who do not tolerate contact lenses. pIOLs implantation indications decreased this last years with the improvement of photoablation profile that allows to treat high ametropia by corneal refractive procedure (LASIK) with an improvement of postoperative quality of vision.

Treatment options for surgical correction of mild to moderate degrees of myopia, astigmatism, and hyperopia include excimer laser photorefractive keratectomy and laser in situ keratomileusis (LASIK). However, for cases of high myopia and hyperopia, these options are limited by a decreased predictability of postoperative results. For this reason, there has been a growing interest in the use of phakic intraocular lenses (pIOLs) to correct refractive errors [1]. pIOL lenses are inserted between the cornea and the natural lens. They are attractive because they preserve accommodation, yield predictable results [1] and have a lower risk of retinal detachment (RD) than in clear lens extraction. Lens designs are of three basic types: anterior chamber IOLs, iris-fixated IOLs, and posterior chamber IOLs that are placed between the iris plane and the natural lens. The implantation of a phakic lens is a major technical refractive surgery, and indications tend to be extended because of the quality of the results outside the domain of high ametropia. It may offer the patient a remarkable functional improvement in terms of quantity and especially quality of vision. However, it may be burdened with complications involving the future of the eye. The choice of surgical approach and type of implant should take into account the notions of efficiency, security as well as reversibility, which should be a major advantage claimed by the technique of refractive surgery [2, 3].

History of Phakic Lenses

In the second half of the 19th century, the fundamentals of refractive surgery were introduced, accompanied by many of the discussions and controversies that still exist in the field today.

Clear lens extraction for the correction of myopia was a concept introduced in the early 1800s, and the technique became increasingly popular from 1850 to 1900 [4].

The first pIOL, an angle-supported pIOL, was described by Strampelli shortly after the introduction of intraocular lenses to correct aphakia in the early 1950s [5]. Later on, Barraquer [6] published the first long-term series of high myopic patients who were implanted with an angle-supported pIOL made of polymethylmethacrylate (PMMA). Both lenses were abandoned due to high incidence of complications. pIOL implantation was reintroduced in 1986 by Fechner and Worst who used a new biconcave iris-fixated IOL to correct high myopia based on modifications made in the iris claw IOLs used in cataract surgery [7–10].

Afterwards, development of a convex-concave lens significantly reduced complications such as glaucoma, endothelial decompensation and iritis.

In 1986, complications that arose from anterior chamber angle-supported pIOLs and iris claw IOLs led to the movement toward the posterior chamber. The rationale was based on the theory that there would be a greater distance between the pIOL and the corneal endothelium. Fyodorov et al. [11] originated the first plate posterior chamber pIOL. They used a one-piece silicone collar button pIOL with a Teflon coat. Encouraging initial results were achieved but problems with cataract formation, uveitis, glaucoma, and decentration led to changes in lens design and type of material to improve biocompatibility. Currently, there are two phakic posterior chamber lenses: the implantable contact lens (ICL) and the phakic refractive lens (PRL).

Then, the 2000s saw the emergence of foldable phakic lenses.

Inclusion and Exclusion Criteria

The following conditions must be fulfilled for phakic lens implantation:
- Contact lens wear is impossible and/or spectacle correction is contraindicated for occupational or psychological reasons
- The age limit is vague: the ideal candidate for placement of a phakic implant is 21–45 years old with an important ametropia, therefore not correctable with excimer laser surgery, or a lower ametropia but associated with LASIK contraindications (thin cornea, corneal scarring, history of corneal surgery)
- Stable refraction for at least 1 year
- Periphery of the retina is healthy or adequately treated
- No history of ocular disease, including glaucoma, cataract, uveitis and macular disease
- Endothelial cell density (ECD) superior to 2,000 cells/mm^2 (specular microscopic examination of the cornea should be performed preoperatively)
- A pupil smaller than 6.0 mm in scotopic luminance (but the reactivity of the pupil seems to be as important as pupil size)
- A deep anterior chamber with an iridocorneal angle >30°
- Lifelong close ophthalmological follow-up should be possible

Today, with the successful results of LASIK for low and moderate myopia, there is a trend to indicate pIOL implantation only in high myopia (9.0 dpt and more), high hyperopia (more than 4 dpt) and high astigmatism (more than 4 dpt).

Exclusion criteria include:
- Previous intraocular surgery
- Endothelial dystrophy
- Opacities of the crystalline lens
- Corneal pathology
- Glaucoma or elevated intraocular pressure (IOP)
- Pigment dispersion syndrome
- Pseudoexfoliation

Table 1. Inclusion and exclusion criteria for pIOL implantation [12]

Inclusion criteria	Exclusion criteria
Age >21 years	Background of active disease in the anterior segment
Stable refraction at least 1 year	Recurrent or chronic uveitis
Ammetropia not correctable with excimer laser surgery	Any form of clinically significant cataract
Unsatisfactory vision with/intolerance of contact lenses or spectacles	Previous corneal or intraocular surgery (to be evaluated)
Iridocorneal angle >30°	IOP >21 mm Hg or glaucoma
cECC >2,300 cells/mm^2: (>2,500 cells/mm^2 if >21 years old, >2,000 if >40 years old)	Preexisting macular degeneration or macular pathology
No anomaly of iris or pupil function	Abnormal retinal condition
Mesopic pupil size <5.0–6.0 mm	Systemic diseases

- Inflammation of the anterior or posterior chamber
- Non-stable ametropia
- History of RD or macular pathology
- Amblyopia and monocularity
- Systemic diseases (e.g. diabetes mellitus, auto-immune disorder, atopia, connective tissue disease) and immunodeficiency
- Anterior chamber depth <3.2 mm
- Pregnancy (transient contraindication) (Table 1)

Preoperative Assessment

The review includes as compulsory information:
- Visual acuity with and without correction
- Manifest and cycloplegic refractions
- Slit-lamp microscope examination
- Applanation tonometry
- Indirect ophthalmoscopy
- Measurement of corneal curvature by keratometry
- Evaluation of corneal thickness, including elevation topography (Orbscan) to investigate a possible keratoconus [13, 14]
- Pupillary diameter measurement with notably pupil diameter in mesopic conditions
- Corneal endothelium analysis by specular microscopic examination (fig. 1)

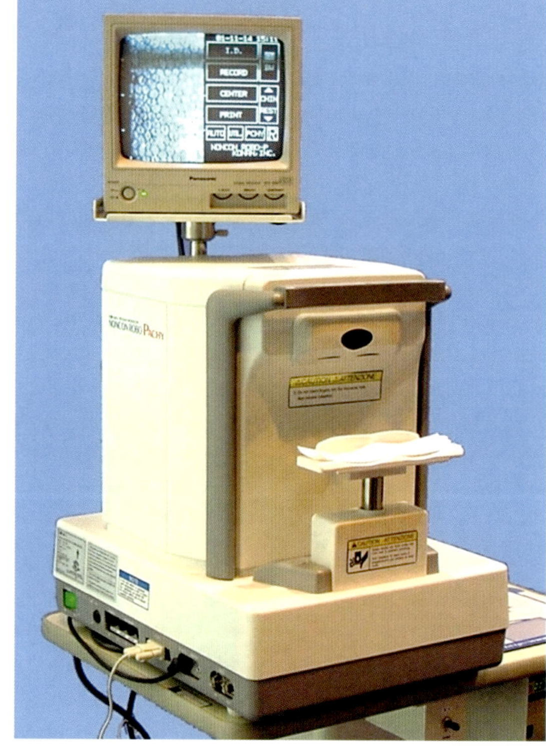

Fig. 1. Specular microscopy.

- The power of the IOL is calculated on the basis of the corneal curvature (K), the anterior chamber depth measured by ultrasonography, and the spectacle correction, by applying a

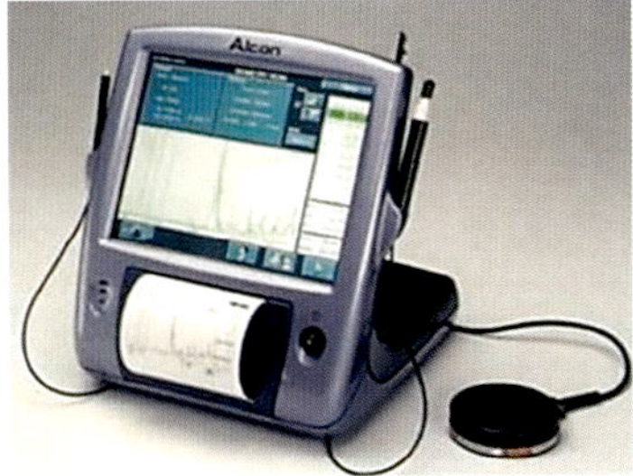

Fig. 2. IOLMaster.

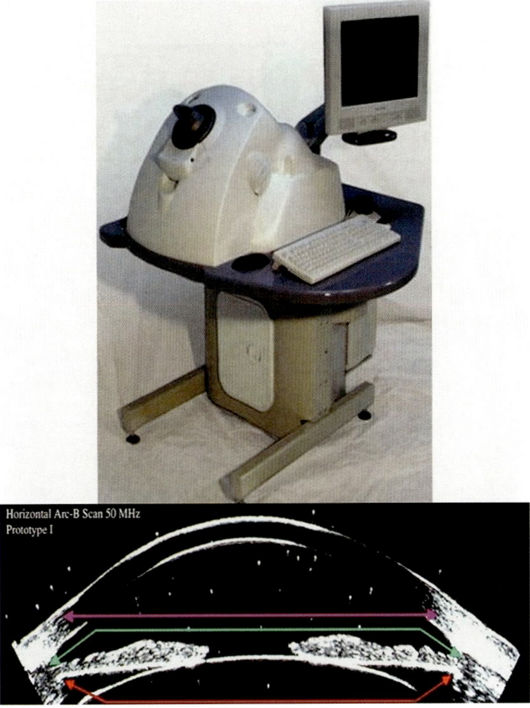

Fig. 3. Ultralink LLC.

special mathematical formula (van der Hei-jde's tables) [15, 16]

- Anterior chamber depth measurements are fundamental because on the one hand, it indicates whether the size of the anterior chamber is sufficient, and on the other hand it is useful for IOL power calculation; it can be obtained by echo ultrasonography in mode A and IOL-Master (fig. 2)
- Anterior chamber diameter measurement with Orbscan provides a measure of white to white diameter which appears to have satisfactory accuracy; emergency technologies such as Ultralink LLC (fig. 3), Pentacam or optical coherence tomography (OCT) [17] (fig. 4) are interesting to explore the anterior segment

The Different Phakic Intraocular Lenses

Angle-Supported Intraocular Lens

Lens Designs
In 1987, Baikoff and Joly [18] developed myopic angle-supported anterior chamber pIOLS. Since then, several generations of this type of lenses appeared such as the ZB, the ZB5M (Domilens Corp.) [19, 20] (fig. 5), the Nuvita MA20 (Bausch & Lomb), the ZSAL-4 (Morcher GmbH) and the safety Flex Phakic 6 H2 (Ophthalmic Innovations International), but they were successively phased out of the market due to unacceptable complica-

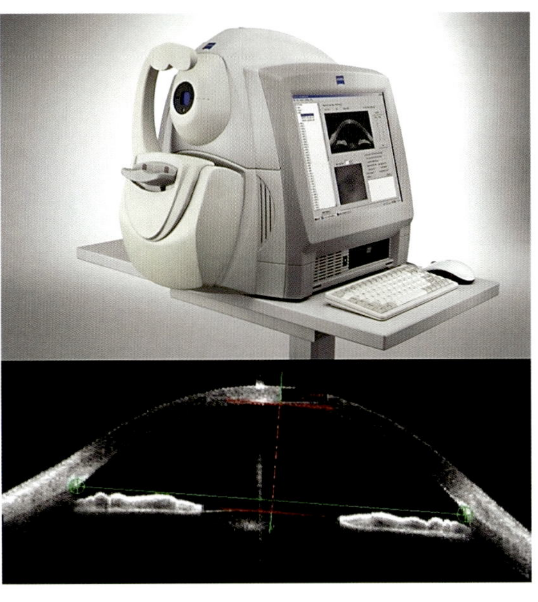

Fig. 4. Visante OCT.

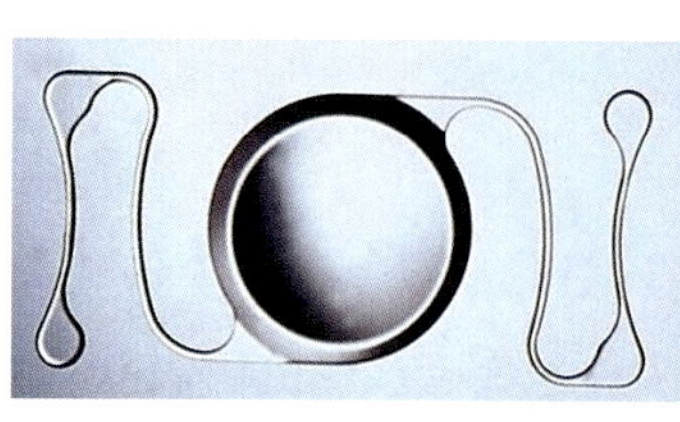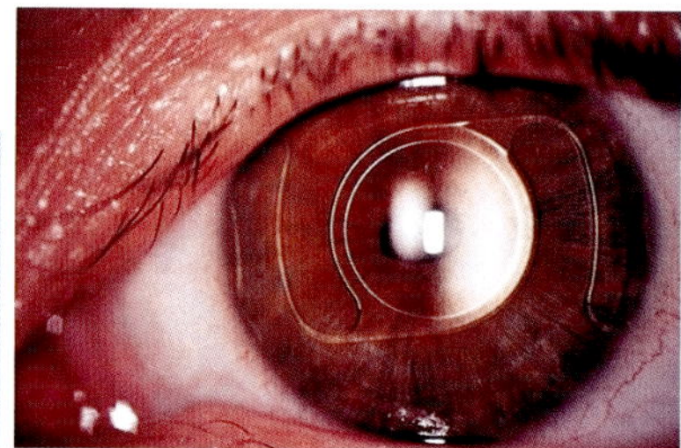

Fig. 5. ZB5M lens.

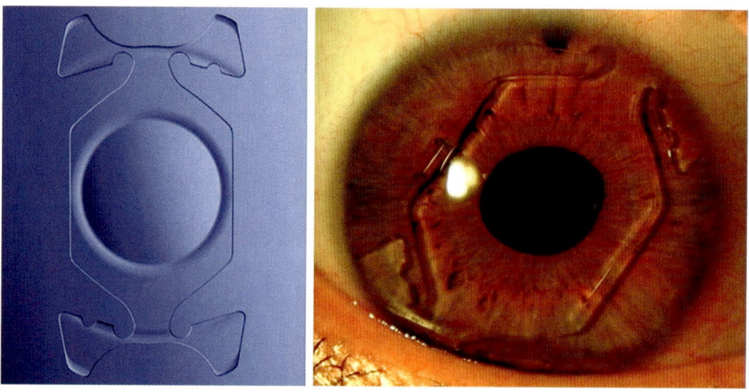

Fig. 6. I-Care lens.

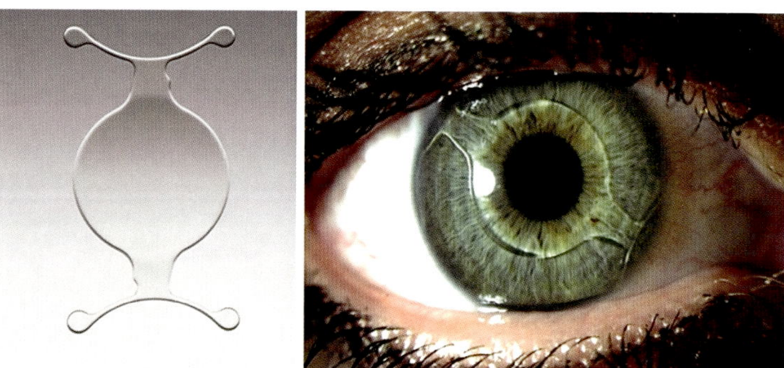

Fig. 7. Acrysof Cachet lens.

tions, including corneal endothelial cell loss, pupil ovalization, glare and halos [21]. It was the same in 2006 and 2008 for the foldable angle-supported lenses such as the GBR Vivarte lens (Ciba Vision-IOLtech) and the I-Care (Corneal Laboratories, Inc.; fig. 6) because of safety concerns related to significant endothelial cell loss [22]. Today, a new anterior chamber angle-supported pIOL has been developed, the Acrysof Cachet (Alcon, Inc.) [23] (fig. 7). The Acrysof Cachet is a single-piece, foldable and a soft acrylic polymeric material with a chemically bonded ultraviolet light-filtering chromophore. Several diameters are available to fit anterior chamber dimensions. Now, it is the last class of this type of lens available on the market.

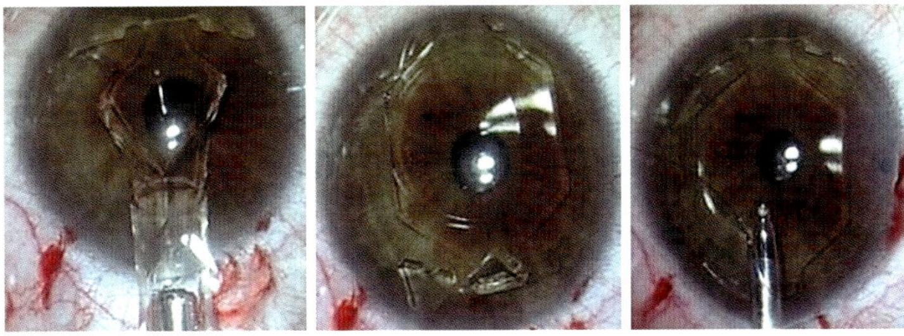

Fig. 8. Angle-supported pIOL implantation.

Surgical Technique

The pIOL size is determined preoperatively by performing the white to white measurement of the anterior chamber diameter. Topical, peribulbar or retrobulbar anesthesia can be used. Iridectomy or iridotomy at the time of surgery is not required.

Before surgery, the pupil is constricted with pilocarpine 2% to protect from possible contact with crystalline lens. It is often completed by injecting acetylcholine (Myochol) in the anterior chamber if pupil constriction is insufficient intraoperatively.

A corneal or limbal tunnel incision of approximately 3.0–3.5 mm is used and usually water tight. The incision is generally oriented temporally, superiorly or along the steepest axis. As of the opening, a great amount of viscoelastic substance is injected to inflate and maintain a deep anterior chamber throughout the procedure. The pIOL is then introduced with a Monarch II or III IOL delivery system (Alcon; fig. 8). After implantation, the viscoelastic is thoroughly removed and a gonioscopic examination is performed to ensure the position and integrity of the pIOL.

The large incisions can be sutured with a single 10-0 nylon.

Complications

They occur mostly with angle-supported pIOLs. The pupil ovalization (fig. 9) was a frequent complication with the previous generation of these lenses. Its incidence increased regularly

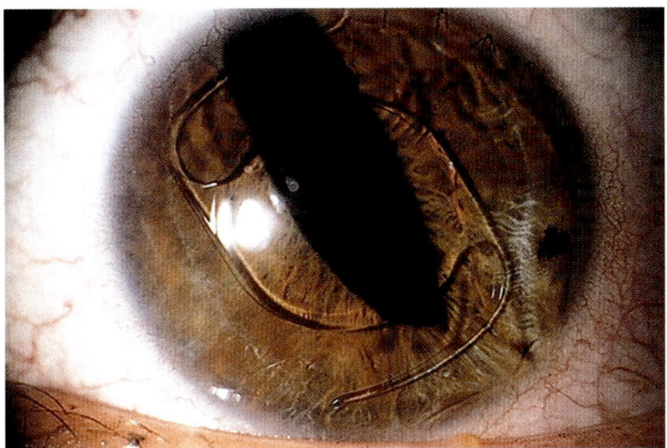

Fig. 9. Pupil ovalization.

with time. It occurred in the large axis of the lens and was associated with a peripheral iris retraction. The ovalization could be induced by the implantation of too large lens or by bad positioning of the haptic. A gross ovalization indicates entrapment of the iris root, and it may become irreversible if the pIOL is not explanted promptly. For these reasons, and the ensuing complications (glare and halos, cosmetic results, iris atrophy), many implants were removed [19, 21]. With the new angle-supported pIOL, the AcrySof Cachet, no case of pupil ovalization was reported [22, 23].

Phakic Intraocular Lens Rotation

A shift of the lens may occur, usually when it is undersized (fig. 10). Pérez-Santonja et al. [24] reported that 43.5% of treated eyes showed a rota-

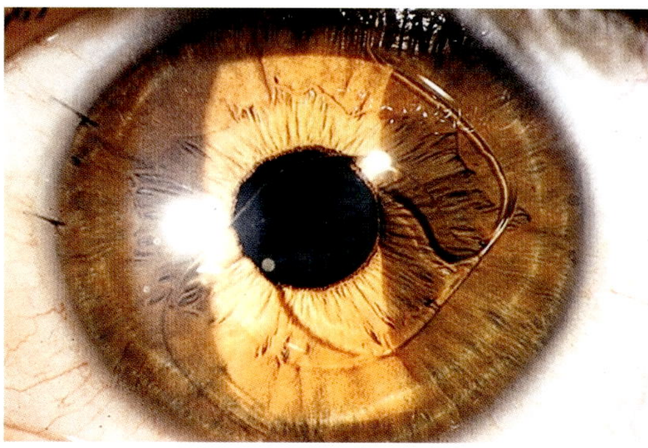

Fig. 10. Shift of the lens.

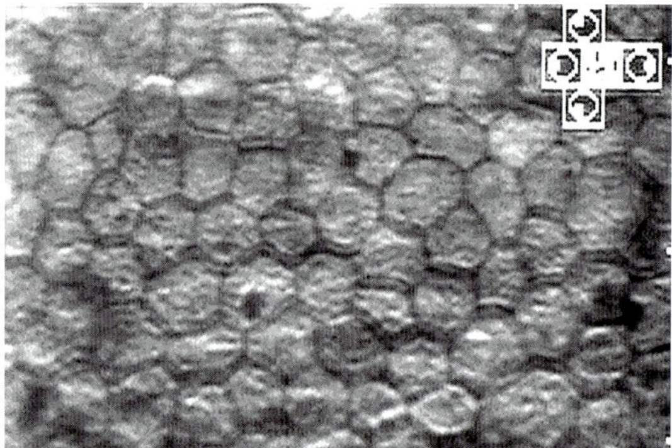

Fig. 11. Endothelial cell loss.

tion, versus only 28.9% with the AcrySof pIOL. However, IOL rotation did not affect the results of the surgery [22].

Endothelial Cell Loss

A permanent implant in the anterior chamber is a continuous risk to progressive corneal endothelial loss with cell abnormalities and marked pleomorphism (fig. 11) [25]. The largest studies were performed with the Baikoff lenses because the first generation of these lenses caused a large cell loss, probably due to contact between the cornea and IOL [25, 26]. The problems with excessive vaulting were minimized with the ZB5M

(angle of 20°). The cumulative endothelial cell loss in the central cornea was significant in the early postoperative period and decreasing after the second postoperative year [27]. Alio et al. [19] reported 7 years of data with similar results; the cumulative endothelial cell loss was 5.53, 6.83, 7.5, 7.78, 8.33, 8.7, and 9.26% for each year of follow-up. In another study, Alio et al. [21] described that endothelial cell loss was a cause of pIOL explantation in 24% of cases. Several generations of anterior chamber pIOL, including new foldable lenses, were withdrawn from the market due to high cell loss (ZB5MF/ZSAL-4, Icare, Vivarte/GBR) [28]. Kohnen et al. [22], in a European multicenter study of the Acrysof foldable anterior chamber pIOL, reported a loss of endothelial cells of 4.8% after 1 year of follow-up. A recent study by Knorz et al. [23] observed that the mean percentage changes in central and peripheral ECD at 6 months were of 3.31 and 2.98%, respectively, and the annualized percentage changes in central ECD and peripheral ECD from 6 months to 3 years were 0.41 and 1.11%, respectively. Another study [29] showed that the Acrysof Cachet pIOL induced a rate of ECD loss consistent with normal age-related changes in the cornea. Kohnen and Klaproth [30] reported a stability of the Acrysof pIOL which maintained an adequate central clearance distance to the corneal endothelium over a period of 3 years. Despite this, a long and regular follow-up is mandatory for each patient.

Cataractogenesis

The analysis of cataractogenesis must also take into account the fact that the majority of these lenses are placed in myopic eyes, which have a natural tendency to develop cataract. The incidence of cataract formation with the new Acrysof pIOL was 2.6%; however, 1% suffered from concurrent ophthalmic disease [22]. Kohnen and Klaproth reported a stable distance between the Acrysof Cachet pIOL and the crystalline lens over a period of 3 years [30].

Glaucoma

Elevation of IOP usually occurs during the early postoperative period and is transient. The most frequent cause is a result of postoperative steroid application in patients who may be sensitive to the medication. Inadequately removed viscoelastic material is an avoidable cause of elevated IOP. It can be prevented with good cleaning of the anterior chamber at the end of surgery. Only a few cases of pupillary block secondary to this surgery have been noted. With Acrysof, iridectomy or iridotomy at the time of surgery are not mandatory. No pupillary block was reported in recent studies [22, 23].

Retinal Detachment

RD is a potential hazard of the pIOL. The reported incidence is very low, but Ruiz-Moreno et al. [31] reported a rate of 4.8% in a large study with ZB5M lenses. It is very difficult to say whether this incidence is induced by the pIOL or myopia. Currently, no case of RD has been reported with the Acrysof pIOL [22, 23].

Visual Outcomes

The results reflect excellent accuracy. Recently, Kohnen et al. [22] reported new European multicenter results with the Acrysof phakic angle-supported IOL. The mean spherical equivalent (SE) was –0.23 dpt at 1 year after operation, and no eye was overcorrected by more than +0.75 dpt. A residual refractive error within ±0.50 dpt was achieved by 72.7% of subjects, and a residual refractive error within ±1.00 dpt was achieved by 95.7%. One year after surgery, 57.8% of subjects achieved an uncorrected distance visual acuity (UCVA) of 20/20 or better, and 99.4% achieved 20/40 or better. 85.7% of subjects achieved a best-corrected visual acuity (BCVA) of 20/20 or better.

Knorz et al. [23], in international multicenter studies, reported a UCVA of 20/40 or better in 97.1% of cases and 20/20 or better in 46.2% of cases with the Acrysof Cachet pIOL. The corrected distance visual acuity was 20/32 or better in 99.0% of patients and 20/20 or better in 80.8% of patients. The mean SE was –0.24 dpt. The residual refractive error was within ±0.50 dpt in 78.8% of subjects and within ±1.00 dpt in 91.3% of subjects.

The angle-supported pIOLs are stable with acceptable safety and predictability to correct ametropia.

Iris-Fixated Intraocular Lens

Lens Designs

Phakic iris-fixated lenses represent an adaptation of Fechner and Worst 'iris claw lens'. Indeed, in 1978 Worst first used this clipping of lens to the iris to correct aphakia after cataract surgery [32]. In 1986, the concept of the claw lens was applied to correct myopia in phakic patients. Initially, the iris claw pIOL for myopia was biconcave (Worst-Fechner biconcave lens) [9].This iris claw lens is fixed to the anterior iris surface by enclavation of a fold of iris tissue into the two diametrically opposed 'claws' of the lens. Despite the good refractive result, a number of cases of endothelial cell loss [19] led to the sec-

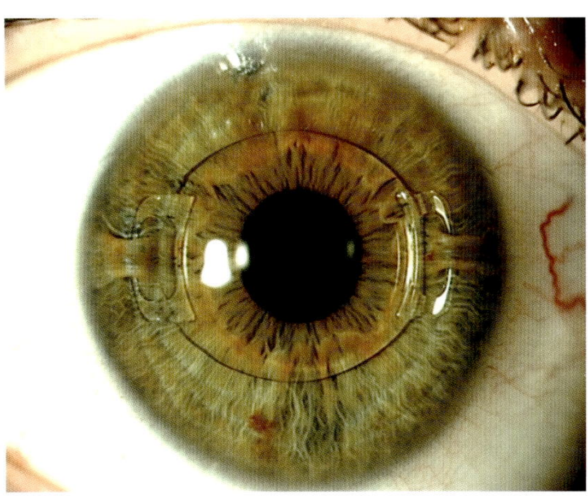

Fig. 12. Artiflex lens.

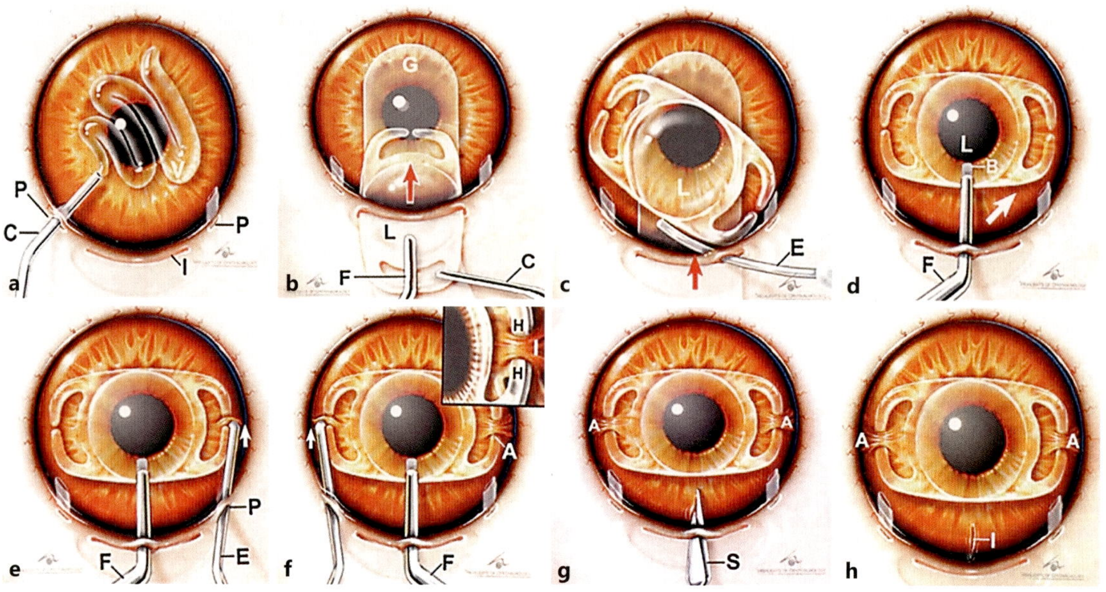

Fig. 13. Iris-fixated pIOL implantation. **a** Viscoelastic injection. **b** Lens insertion. **c** Lens rotation. **d** Lens centration. **e** Lens enclavation. **f** Lens enclavation. **g** Peripheral iridectomy. **h** Viscoelastic removal.

ond generation of this phakic implant in 1991 under the name Artisan™ (Ophtec BV; fig. 12), which then replaced the name 'iris claw' or Worst. The design of this lens was modified into a convex-concave design to increase the distance between the pIOL and the corneal endothelium. The anterior convexity improves the optical quality of this lens by reducing its prismatic effect. The posterior face ensures optimal space in front of the natural lens and prevents aqueous flow blockage. Made of PMMA, these lenses are available in two different diameters, 5.5 and 6 mm, since 1997 to correct myopia. Following the excellent results of the myopic Artisan, a configuration for hyperopia was introduced in 1995. The Artisan toric lens (fig. 1) is available since 2001 to correct astigmatism, and combines a spherical anterior face and spherocylindrical posterior face [33, 34]. A foldable version of the iris-fixated lens marketed under the name Artiflex™ (Ophtec BV)/Veriflex™ (Abbott Medical Optics, Inc.; fig. 2) is available since 2005 [35]. In 2009, a final version of foldable toric lens to correct astigmatism has been marketed.

Surgical Technique

The surgical technique is shown in figure 13. Preoperative miosis is required to protect the crystalline lens. It can be completed by injecting acetylcholine (Miochol) in the anterior chamber at the beginning of surgery. Miosis forms a protective shield for the natural lens during the insertion and fixation of the iris claw.

More patients are operated on an outside basis. General anesthesia is recommended during the learning curve. Once the surgical technique is mastered, local anesthesia can be used if the total immobility of the globe and the eyelids can be achieved; Whatever the type of anesthesia, preoperative bulbar compression is suggested by some surgeons in order to lower the ocular pressure to lower the risk of iris prolapse.

Various incision techniques can be used: clear corneal or scleral tunnel incision superiorly. The size of the incision depends on the diameter of the optical zone, 5 or 6 mm for rigid lens and tunneled to be watertight from 3.2 to 3.5 mm for foldable lens. The next step is the achievement of two small vertical incisions of at least 1.1 mm at 10 o'clock and 2 o'clock, directed toward the enclavation area. The viscoelastic substance is injected through one of the puncture incisions to create a deep anterior chamber. The pIOL is introduced with the Artisan fixation forceps into the anterior chamber. Then the pIOL is rotated 90°. Centration and fixation of the IOL is the most critical step; pupil is used as a reference for centration. Fixation of the IOL is performed by gently creating an iris fold under the claw with an enclavation hook and consequently entrapping the iris fold into the claw. It is also possible to use holding forceps; in this case, the incisions are made in front of enclavation place. A prophylactic iridectomy or iridotomy must be performed to prevent pupillary block. Wound suture is started prior to removal of the viscoelastic material.

Particularities of the Toric Lens

A careful preoperative biomicroscopic examination of the iris with the patient sitting up (to avoid rotation of the globe) is necessary.

Particularities of the Artiflex Lens

The Artiflex foldable lens is inserted using a spatula through a small incision. For the enclavation, special curved forceps which hold the base of the PMMA haptic are used.

Complications

Anterior Chamber Inflammation

There may be correlation between the incidence of some complications and the experience of the surgeon. Rare cases of exudative iritis were described during the early period of the surgeon's learning curve, probably due to repeated traumatic attempts of iridal incarceration [7, 36, 37]. The iris

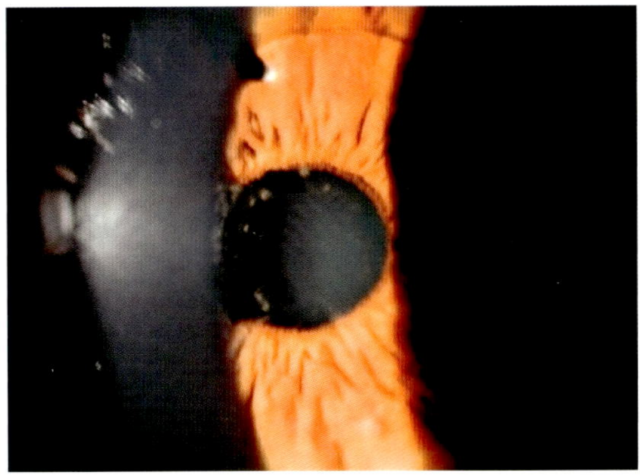

Fig. 14. Pigmented deposits.

fixation could induce a prolonged breakdown of the blood-aqueous barrier and consequently a chronic subclinical inflammation. Studies using laser flare-cell meter showed contradictory results. Pérez-Santonja et al. [38, 39], using a laser flare-cell meter, detected chronic subclinical inflammation between 1 and 2 years postoperatively. Conversely, Fechner et al. [36] reported no more inflammation than after a cataract extraction with posterior chamber implantation. Malecaze et al. [40, 41], in their studies did not find any significant increase of flare values. Finally, iris angiography did not show vascular leaks in some studies [36, 37].

Pigment Dispersion/Lens Deposits

Pigment cells are occasionally visible on the pIOL optic in the early postoperative period from surgical trauma [42–44] (fig. 14). Convex iris could be more prone to develop pigment dispersion [42]. These pigment precipitates differ from non-pigment precipitates reported after implantation with silicone-foldable lens [45] (fig. 15). The adhesiveness of the material has been implicated. We have not found, in our experience, significant intraocular inflammation associated with the presence of non-pigment precipitates on the lens [41].

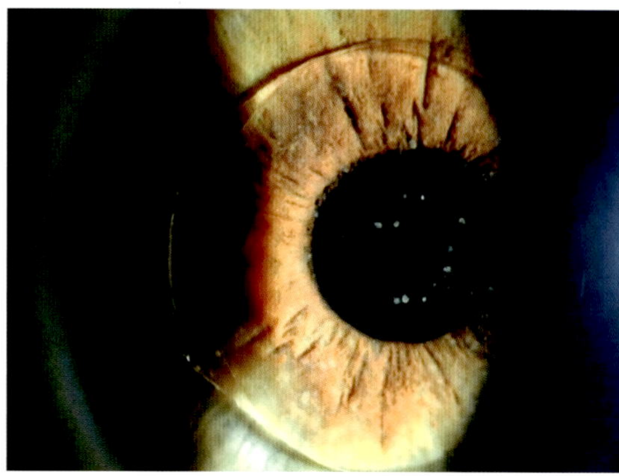

Fig. 15. Nonpigmented deposits.

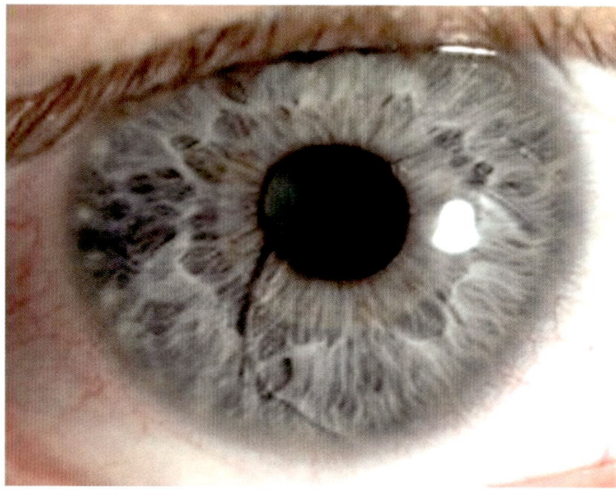

Fig. 16. Traumatic disenclavation.

Glaucoma

Only rare cases of transient ocular hypertension have been reported [37]. Postoperative glaucoma can be corticosteroid induced, and usually resolves after discontinuation of steroidal therapy. Pupil block glaucoma is a complication of non-functional peripheral iridectomy. Transient ocular hypertension can also occur if the viscoelastic material has not been adequately removed.

Iris Atrophy/Dislocation

Several authors reported iris atrophy on fixation sites due to the imperfect enclavation. IOL dislocation is usually due to an insufficient amount of iris tissue fold through the claw and is usually provoked by an ocular trauma (fig. 16).

Endothelial Cell Loss

Risk of endothelial cell loss after implantation with an iris-fixated lens may be related to initial surgical trauma but also postoperatively, the geometry of the lens as well as the depth of the anterior chamber. The literature data are contradictory and difficult to compare because studies sometimes include lenses from different generations [46–53]. According to Fechner et al. [10], significant progressive endothelial cell loss was observed in 13.4% of eyes implanted between 1986 and 1991, and a projected 8-year follow-up resulted in a decrease in 27% of eyes with biconcave lenses. It was a major reason behind the design change to the convex-concave shape of the Artisan myopia lens. Güell et al. [46] in a European multicenter study on 399 eyes implanted with iris claw pIOLs reported an average endothelial cell loss of 6.99% (n = 319) at 3 years.

Visual Outcomes

Several studies have shown that concerning high myopia the results are satisfactory in terms of the refractive outcome. In the earlier series of Fechner et al. [7] (62 eyes; preoperative SE –7.0 to –28.0 dpt), 63% of eyes were within 1.0 dpt correction. None deviated more than 20% from the predicted correction. In a series of 78 eyes (range –6.0 to –28.0 dpt) reported by Landesz et al. [54], 67.9% had a postoperative refraction within ±1.0 dpt of emmetropia. A study by Maloney et al. [55] confirmed that the Verisyse lens (Abbott Medical Optics, Inc.) is an accurate method for the correction of high myopia with 90% of eyes within 1 dpt of attempted correction. Malecaze et al. [56], in his unpublished series of 25 eyes (mean SE –13.43 dpt, range –8.00

to –17.25 dpt) implanted with the Artisan myopia lens (Ophtec BV), found a 52% (13 eyes) and 84% (21 eyes) predictability value for 0.5 dpt or less and 1.0 dpt or less of aimed postoperative UCVA, respectively. Efficacy, defined as the ratio between postoperative UCVA and preoperative BCVA, was 0.80 in his series. Visual recovery was rapid since mean UCVA was 0.46 ± 0.22 dpt on the first postoperative day. More recently, Menezo et al. [57] reported that the mean UCVA before surgery was 0.014 and the mean BCVA before surgery was 0.52 in the Artisan group. Coullet et al. [41] reported that the percentage of eyes with UCVA of >20/40 was 51.6% (16/31 patients) for Artisan-treated eyes and 77.4% (24/31 patients) for Artiflex-treated eyes one year after surgery. Dick et al. [35] in a series of 290 eyes implanted with the foldable Artiflex pIOL, found after 2 years an UCVA of 20/40 or better in 97.2% of eyes and a BSCVA of 20/40 or better in all eyes.

Recent studies by Alio et al. [58], Saxena et al. [59] and Guell et al. [46], have reported that implantation with the Artisan/Verisyse for correcting high hyperopia leads to accurate refractive results with no significant loss of vision.

Two recent multicenter studies [60, 61] have proven the remarkable results of the Verisyse toric lens for the correction of ametropia with high astigmatism. The quasi totality of the eye was within 1 dpt of emmetropia, and there was a reduction in the preoperative astigmatism with an average magnitude of residual postoperative astigmatism of <0.8 dpt.

Very rarely, visual symptoms such as double contour are reported. Postoperative glare and halos usually disappear gradually [37].

Posterior Chamber Phakic Intraocular Lens

Lens Designs
In 1993, Zaldivar, Davidorf, and Oscherow began implanting a plate posterior chamber pIOL

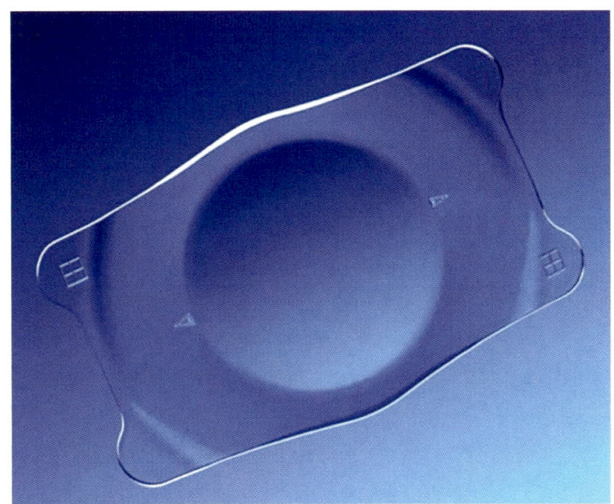

Fig. 17. STAAR Visian ICL.

(STAAR Surgical ICL) [62]. This lens design was modified from the one Fyodorov originated in 1986 [63] using a one-piece silicone collar-button pIOL with a 500- to 600-nm Teflon coat. Incorporation of a porcine collagen-HEMA copolymer into the lens material has improved the lens's biocompatibility. Phase I trials by the Food and Drug Administration were approved in February 1997 for the treatment of hyperopia with this posterior chamber pIOL [64].

Two models of posterior chamber pIOLs are currently available:

- The STARR surgical ICL (fig. 17) is made of a collagen copolymer, a compound combining acrylic and porcine collagen. The polymer material is soft, elastic, and hydrophilic. The posterior surface is concave. The current model, the Visian ICL V4, is a rectangular single-piece IOL. The optical zone diameter of myopic lenses varies between 4.5 and 5.5 mm according to the power required. For hyperopic lenses, it is 5.5 mm. Available powers are –3 to –23 dpt for myopic lenses, and +3 to +22 dpt for hyperopic lenses with an added positive cylinder of +1 to +6 dpt for toric ICLs correcting myopia [65]. The posterior surface is concave in order to vault over the anterior capsule. This implant is placed in the ciliary sulcus. It is intended for the treatment of myopia, hyperopia and astigmatism.

- The CIBA PRL (fig. 18) is made from an ultrathin silicon polymer. This material is soft, elastic, and hydrophobic. The width is 6.0 mm; two lengths are available for myopic lenses: 10.8 or 11.3 mm and one for hyperopic lenses: 10.6 mm. Available powers are –3 to –20 for myopic lenses, and +3 to +15 for hyperopic lenses. The lens has no anatomical fixation sites; it is supposed to move unaided into a centered position inside the posterior chamber spaces without exerting pressure on the ciliary structures, the zonula in particular [66]. It is not in contact with the anterior capsule of the crystalline lens: it 'floats'.

Surgical Technique

The surgical technique is presented in figure 19. A combination of mydriatic topical medications (tropicamide 1%, phenylephrine 2.5% or similar) is applied serially, beginning 1 h before surgery. The anesthesia method (general anesthesia, peribulbar injection or topical anesthesia) is based on patient and surgeon preference.

Two weeks before surgery, laser iridotomies are performed. Two peripheral superior iridotomies are placed 80° apart to avoid the possibility of iridotomy occlusion by the haptics of the implant. Otherwise, a surgical iridectomy will be performed at the time of implantation.

A temporal corneal tunnel (width 3.2 mm, length 1.75–2 mm) is created. Viscoelastic (ideally methylcellulose) is injected into the anterior chamber. The implant can be injected by different techniques:

- With an injector [67]. The IOL is positioned in the lens insertion cartridge under direct visualization with the operating microscope. In the absence of a soft-tip injector, a small silicone sponge can be placed to protect the IOL from the hard injector arm. Because IOL insertion in the cartridge is complicated and time-consuming, it must be performed before the incision is made. The injector tip is placed in the tunnel, and the lens is injected into the anterior chamber. As the IOL unfolds slowly, its progression must be controlled to ensure proper orientation.

- With forceps [67]. The IOL is easy to fold between the jaws of MacPherson forceps. The tip of the forceps is introduced into the entrance of the tunnel. Then another MacPherson forceps held in the operator's other hand is used to grasp the sides of the implant. The first forceps are opened; they re-grasp the IOL a little further, and push it slowly. By repeating these maneuvers with the forceps, the IOL moves into the tunnel and can unfold in a controlled manner. The tip of the forceps must never enter into the anterior chamber so as to avoid contact with the crystalline lens.

While the IOL unfolds, its proper orientation must be checked. Then, each foot plate is placed one after the other beneath the iris with a specially designed, flat, non-polished manipulator, without placing pressure on the crystalline lens. It is important to avoid touching the optic of an ICL in the middle, as this is the thinnest part. Then, the viscoelastic is removed with gentle irrigation-aspiration, and acetylcholine chloride is injected. An iridectomy or iridotomy must be performed to prevent pupillary block. Finally, the wound is hydrated.

The procedure for the PRL is similar, the lens is grasped by the special forceps designed to

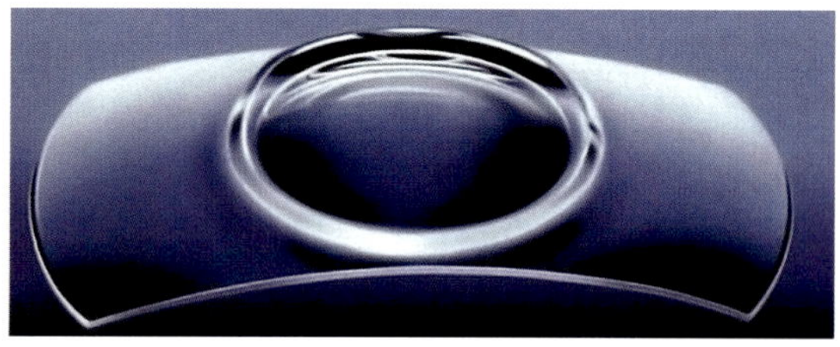

Fig. 18. CIBA PRL.

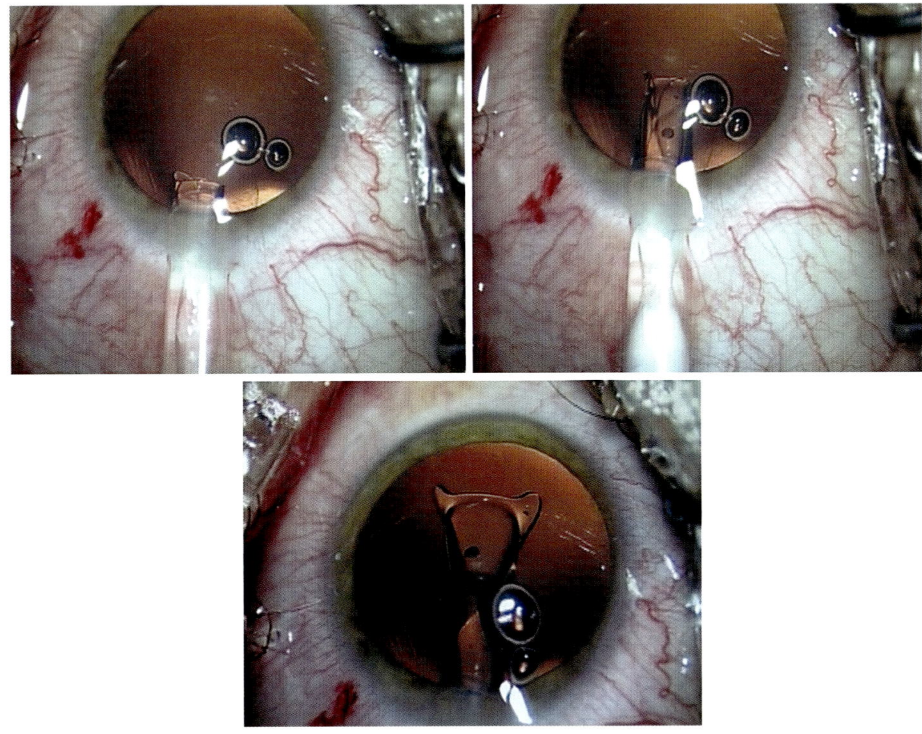

Fig. 19. Implantation of the STAAR ICL.

prevent damage on the optical zone (Dementiev forceps) or it is inserted with an injector system.

Complications
Pigment Dispersion and Elevated Intraocular Pressure
A pigmentary reaction was first reported by Asseto et al. [68]. Pigment deposits on the periphery of the ICL optic (fig. 20) is constant 1 year after surgery, but it has no visual consequence. In two cases [64], pigmentary deposits that were not present preoperatively were seen in the angle in association with elevated IOP. According to Zaldivar et al. [62], this is a non-progressive pigmentation.

Although contact and rubbing of the optic shoulder against the posterior surface of the iris

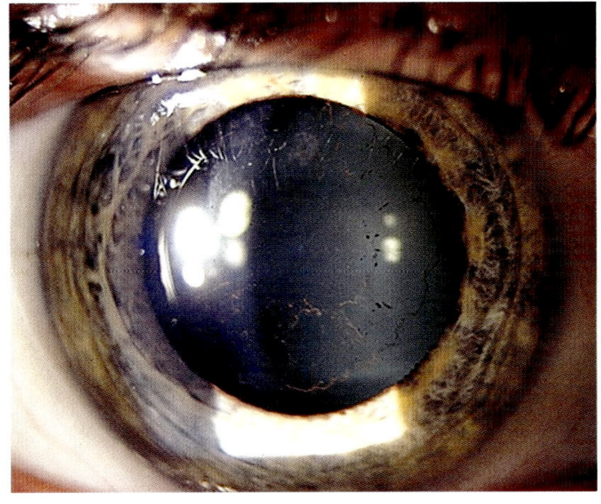

Fig. 20. Pigment deposits on the IOL.

have been shown using ultrasound biomicroscopy [69–71], some of the pigment dispersion [69] may be partly surgically induced by YAG iridotomies and trauma of the iris during implantation [70]. Pigmentary dispersion can be of some concern because highly myopic eyes are, by their nature, at increased risk of developing glaucoma [67].

Elevation of IOP can result from several mechanisms, including postoperative use of topical corticosteroids, narrowing of the angle (demonstrated by ultrasound biomicroscopy studies [69], especially in hyperopic eyes), and pigmentary deposits in the angle [64]. Several recent studies do not report a significant increase in IOP [57, 72, 73]. In contrast, other authors have reported an increase in IOP and some cases of secondary glaucoma after implantation [74, 75].

Endothelial Cell Loss
Although endothelial cell loss is a major concern with anterior chamber IOLs, it does not seem to be an issue with posterior chamber pIOLs. Fyodorov et al. [11] reported a mean decrease in ECD of 5% with their silicone posterior chamber pIOL, and Asseto et al. [68] found a mean endothelial cell loss of 4% with the STAAR IOL. Arné and Lesueur [76] noted a mean endothelial cell loss of 2.1% 3 months after surgery with the same pIOL (2.3% at 6 months, 2% at 1 year, and 2% at 2 years). Endothelial cell loss never exceeded 3.8% at 1 year [67, 76]. Dejaco-Ruhswurm et al. [77] evaluated the long-term endothelial cell change in phakic eyes after implantation of the STAAR IOL; they noted a rapid loss until 1 year postoperatively, after which the rate of loss was no longer statistically significant. This absence of chronic ongoing endothelial loss has also been confirmed by more recent studies [77, 78]. Kamiya et al. [79] reported corneal endothelial cell loss of 3.7% at 4 years after ICL implantation.

Cataractogenesis
Cataract formation (fig. 21) is one of the most crucial concerns for the future of posterior cham-

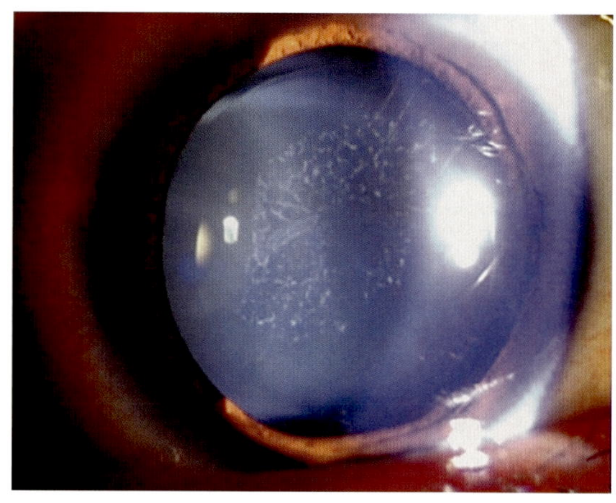

Fig. 21. Cataractogenesis.

ber pIOLs [67]. Trindade and Pereira [80] reported a case of significant cataract formation 6 months after uneventful ICL implantation. Fink et al. [81] reported on the occurrence of lens opacification in 3 eyes of 2 patients. Arné and al. [76] observed 2 cases (3.4%) of anterior subcapsular opacities; one required removal of the ICL followed by phacoemulsification and posterior chamber IOL implantation. Lackner et al. [82] reported on subcapsular anterior opacifications of the crystalline lens in 25 of 75 eyes (33.3%) that received an ICL. A meta-analysis of cataract development after posterior chamber pIOL surgery published by Chen et al. [83] found that 223 of 1,210 eyes developed new-onset cataract. The incidence of cataract formation was 8.5% for the ICL pIOL and 3.6% for the PRL. The recently published Food and Drug Administration [84] study showed an incidence of 2.1% of anterior subcapsular opacities with the ICL V4 model.

Cataract may form as a result of trauma to the crystalline lens during the implantation procedure. However, in most reported cases, the implantation was non-traumatic. Contact between the ICL and the central area of the crystalline lens is considered as the cause of cataract formation [67]. Examination by ultrasound biomicroscopy and Scheimpflug camera [71, 72, 76, 81] can demonstrate this contact in case of insufficient vault. A study using very high-frequency ultrasound on 2 eyes implanted with new posterior chamber pIOLs failed to show any contact between the implant and the natural lens, even during accommodation and light reflex [85]. The choice of a large implant appears necessary to obtain a greater axial vault, along with a larger space between the ICL and the central part of the crystalline lens. However, an excessive vault pushes the iris forward and favors narrowing of the angle, increases contact between the ICL and the posterior surface of the iris, and, consequently, pigmentary dispersion. Excessive vault may also induce contact between the haptics of the ICL and the periphery of the crystalline lens. Metabolic disturbances induced by the material of the implant may also be partially responsible for cataract formation.

The treatment of cataract in patients implanted with posterior chamber pIOLs is not difficult. Explantation of the ICL is easily performed through the same size primary clear corneal incision. Phacoemulsification and posterior chamber IOL implantation can be done in a routine fashion.

Visual Outcomes
In the series of phakic implantation in myopic eyes by Zaldivar et al. [62], the preoperative BCVA was 20/40 or better in 80% and 20/20 or better in 5% of the eyes. Postoperatively, UCVA was 20/40 or better in 93% and 20/20 or better in 19% of the eyes. A gain of two or more lines of postoperative BCVA was attained in 36% of the cases; 7% of the eyes lost one line, 0.8% lost two lines.

In the series reported by Arné and al. [76], the mean preoperative BCVA was 0.57 and the mean postoperative UCVA and BCVA were 0.40 and 0.71, respectively. The postoperative UCVA was better than the preoperative BCVA in 15.5% of the cases, unchanged in 15.5% and worse in 68.9% of the eyes. The mean efficacy index (ratio of postoperative UCVA to preoperative BCVA) was 0.84. Safety, calculated as the ratio between postoperative and preoperative values was 1.46.

Menezo et al. [57] reported that the mean UCVA before surgery was 0.03 in the STAAR group, and 18 months after surgery the UCVA was 0.50. The mean BCVA before surgery was 0.49, whereas at 18 months, it improved and was 0.78.

Pallikaris et al. [66], after implantation of PRLs in myopic eyes, noted an improvement of BCVA from 0.70 ± 0.24 to 0.85 ± 0.24.

In the series of myopic and hyperopic patients implanted with PRL by Hoyos et al. [86], lines of BCVA were gained in 65% of the myopic eyes. No eye lost one line of BCVA. In the hyperopic group, one eye gained one line of BCVA and one eye lost one line.

Boxer et al. [87], reported that postoperative UCVA of 20/20 or better and 20/25 or better in the Visian ICL group was 67 and 96%, respectively. A gain of one or two lines of postoperative best spectacle-corrected visual acuity was obtained in 40 and 10% of the cases, respectively.

Good efficacy and predictability have been demonstrated in all studies on posterior chamber phakic lenses for treatment of high myopias. The marked gain in postoperative BCVA compared with preoperative spectacle BCVA in high myopes is largely due to elimination of the spectacle-induced image reduction.

Conversely, only 8% of the hyperopic eyes operated on by Davidorf et al. [88] demonstrated a gain in postoperative BCVA compared to the preoperative spectacle BCVA. In this series, 7 of 24 eyes (29%) lost one or more lines of postoperative spectacle BCVA. This is explained by the loss of magnification induced by the surgery. Also, 4% of the eyes lost two or more lines of spectacle BCVA due to postoperative glaucoma.

In the series by Koivula et al. [73], the difference between pre- and postoperative UCVA results was significant, but the difference between 3 months and 1 year was not significant and the results were similar to BCVA.

Indication of the Model of Phakic Intraocular Lenses

In the absence of contraindications, pIOL implantation is the best approach in young patients with high refractive errors and in those who have a contraindication to a corneal refractive procedure. Advantages are that pIOL implantation preserves corneal architecture, asphericity and accommodation. pIOLs are divided into 3 types described above. Each design has its own features, selection criteria, surgical technique, results and complications. The principal risk of angle-supported IOLs and iris-fixated IOLs is the loss of corneal endothelial cells or damage to the endothelial integrity. Therefore, a long-term follow-up of each patient with an anterior chamber pIOL is mandatory to detect patients who have significant damage to the endothelium and explant the pIOL whenever clinically necessary. Implantation of anterior chamber pIOLs is particularly indicated in young patients or in those with deep anterior chamber. The main complication of posterior chamber pIOLs is anterior subcapsular cataract formation. Thus, this site of implantation of phakic implants is preferred in older patients or in those with narrow anterior chamber.

Conclusion

pIOL implantation for the correction of myopia and hyperopia seems to be an effective and predictable alternative to keratorefractive surgery, particularly for high refractive errors. Currently, two different surgical refractive alternatives are predominantly used: the corneal refractive procedure (LASIK) and the intraocular lens surgery. These techniques are precise, reproducible and produce similar successful optical results.

The choice between the two techniques is still a matter of debate because they do not have the same advantages and disadvantages. A major concern with LASIK is its risk of corneal ectasia, whereas with pIOL, endothelial cell loss or cataractogenesis are feared.

Today, with new ablation profiles, the LASIK technique can treat myopia up to –9 dpt, high astigmatism and hyperopia up to +4.5 dpt. Therefore, pIOLs have fewer indications than previously.

All things considered, when trying to make the best choice for a patient with moderately high myopia, the individual parameters of the cornea and the anterior chamber depth must first be taken into account.

References

1 Yoo S: Phakic IOL implantation: comparison with keratorefractive surgical procedures; in Azar DT (ed): Intraocular Lenses in Cataract and Refractive Surgery. Philadelphia, WB Saunders, 2001, pp 239–244.

2 Saragoussi JJ, Arné JL, Colin J, Montard M: Chirurgie refractive. Rapport Société Française d'Ophtalmologie. Masson, Paris, 2001.

3 Azard DT: Intraocular Lenses in Cataract and Refractive Surgery, Philadelphia, WB Saunders, 2001.

4 Seiler T: Clear lens extraction in the 19th century – an early demonstration of premature dissemination. J Refract Surg 1999;15:70–73.

5 Strampelli B: Sopportabilita di lenti acriliche in camera anteriore nella afachia e nei vizi di refrazione. Ann Oftalmol Clin Oculist 1954;80:5–82.

6 Barraquer JI: Anterior chamber plastic lenses. Results of and conclusions from five years experience. Trans Ophthalmol Soc UK 1959;79:393–424.

7 Fechner PU, van der Heijde GL, Worst JG: The correction of myopia by lens implantation into phakic eyes. Am J Ophthalmol 1989;107:659–663.

8 Los LI, Worst JG: Implant surgery. Something old and something new. Doc Ophthalmol 1990;75:377–390.

9 Worst JGF, van der Veen G, Los LI: Refractive surgery for high myopia. The Worst-Fechner biconcave iris claw lens. Doc Ophthalmol 1990;75:335–341.

10 Fechner PU, Haubitz I, Wichmann W, Wulff K: Worst-Fechner biconcave minus power phakic iris-claw lens. J Refract Surg 1999;15:93–105.

11 Fyodorov SN, Zuev VK, Tumanyan ER: Modern approach to the stagewise complex surgical therapy of high myopia. Transactions of International Symposium of IOL Implantation and Refractive Surgery. Moscow, RS-FSP Ministry of Health, 1987, pp 27427–27429.

12 Güell JL, Morral M, Kook D, Kohnen T: Phakic intraocular lenses. J Cataract Refract Surg 2010;36:1976–1993.

13 Liu Z, Huang AJ, Pflugfelder SC: Evaluation of corneal thickness and topography in normal eyes using the Orbscan corneal topography system. Br J Ophthalmol 1999;83:774–778.

14 van der Heijde GL, Fechner PU, Worst JGF: Optische Konsequenzen der Implantation einer negativen Intraokularlinse bei myopen Patienten. Klin Mbl Augenheilk 1988;193:99–102.

15 van der Heijde GL: Some optical aspects of implantation of an IOL in a myopic eye. Eur J Implant Ref Surg 1989;1:245–248.

16 Sedaghat MR, Daneshvar R, Kargozar A, Derakhshan A, Daraei M: Comparison of central corneal thickness measurement using ultrasonic pachymetry, rotating Scheimpflug camera, and scanning-slit topography. Am J Ophthalmol 2010;150:780–789.

17 Lizzi FL, Coleman DJ: History of ophthalmic ultrasound. J Ultrasound Med 2004;23:1255–1266.

18 Baikoff G, Joly P: Correction chirurgicale de la forte myopie par les implants phakes de chambre antérieure. Concept et résultats. Bull Soc Belge Ophtalmol 1989;233:109–125.

19 Alió JL, de la Hoz F, Peréz-Santonja JJ, Ruiz-Moreno JM, Quesada JA: Phakic anterior chamber lenses for the correction of myopia: a 7-year cumulative analysis of complications in 263 cases. Ophthalmology 1999;106:458–466.

20 Alió JL, de la Hoz F, Ruiz-Moreno JM, Salem TF: Cataract surgery in highly myopic eyes corrected by phakic anterior chamber angle-supported lenses. J Cataract Refract Surg 2000;26:1303–1311.

21 Alió JL, Abdelrahman AM, Javaloy J, Iradier MT, Ortuño V: Angle-supported anterior chamber phakic intraocular lens explantation causes and outcome. Ophthalmology 2006;113:2212–2213.

22 Kohnen T, Knorz MC, Cochener B, Gerl RH, Arné J-L, Colin J, et al: AcrySof phakic angle-supported intraocular lens for the correction of moderate-to-high myopia: one-year results of a multicenter European study. Ophthalmology 2009; 116:1314–1321, 1321.e1–e3.

23 Knorz MC, Lane SS, Holland SP: Angle-supported phakic intraocular lens for correction of moderate to high myopia: three-year interim results in international multicenter studies. J Cataract Refract Surg 2011;37:469–480.

24 Pérez-Santonja JJ, Alió JL, Jiménez-Alfaro I, Zato MA: Surgical correction of severe myopia with an angle-supported phakic intraocular lens. J Cataract Refract Surg 2000;26:1288–1302.

25 Mimouni F, Colin J, Koff V, et al: Damage to the corneal endothelium from anterior chamber intraocular lenses in phakic myopic eyes. Refract Corneal Surg 1991;7:277–281.

26 Bour T, Piquot X, Pospisil A, et al: Repercussions endothéliales de l'implant myopique de chambre antérieure ZB au cours de la première année: etude prospective avec analyse statistique. J Fr Ophtalmol 1991;14: 633–641.

27 Baikoff G, Arne JL, Bokobza Y, et al: Angle-fixated anterior chamber phakic intraocular lens for myopia of –7 to –19 diopters (see comments). J Refract Surg 1998;14:282–293.

28 Gierek-Ciaciura S, Gierek-Lapinska A, Ochalik K, Mrukwa-Kominek E: Correction of high myopia with different phakic anterior chamber intraocular lenses: ICARE angle-supported lens and Verisyse iris-claw lens. Graefes Arch Clin Exp Ophthalmol 2007;245:1–7.

29 Lane SS, Waycaster C: Correction of high myopia with a phakic intraocular lens: interim analysis of clinical and patient-reported outcomes. J Cataract Refract Surg 2001;37:1426–1433.

30 Kohnen T, Klaproth OK: Three-year stability of an angle-supported foldable hydrophobic acrylic phakic intraocular lens evaluated by Scheimpflug photography. J Cataract Refract Surg 2010;36: 1120–1126.

31 Ruiz-Moreno JM, Alio JL, Perez-Santonja JJ: Retinal detachment in phakic eyes with anterior chamber intraocular lenses to correct severe myopia. Am J Ophthalmol 1999;127:270–275.

32 Worst JG: Iris claw lens. J Am Intraocul Implant Soc 1980;6:166–167.

33 Tehrani M, Dick HB: Iris-fixated toric phakic intraocular lens: three-year follow-up. J Cataract Refract Surg 2006;32:1301–1306.

34 Alió JL, Mulet ME, Gutiérrez R, Galal A: Artisan toric phakic intraocular lens for correction of astigmatism. J Refract Surg 2005;21:324–331.

35 Dick HB, Budo C, Malecaze F, Güell JL, Marinho AA, Nuijts RM, Luyten GP, Menezo JL, Kohnen T: Foldable Artiflex phakic intraocular lens for the correction of myopia: two-year follow-up results of a prospective European multicenter study. Ophthalmology 2009;116:671–677.

36 Fechner PU, Strobel J, Wichmann W: Correction of myopia by implantation of a concave worst-iris claw lens into phakic eyes. Refract Corneal Surg 1991;7: 286–298.

37 Menezo JL, Avino JA, Cisneros AL, Rodriguez-Salvador V, Martiez-Costa R: Iris claw phakic intraocular lens for high myopia. J Refract Surg 1997;13:545–555.

38 Pérez-Santonja JJ, Bueno JL, Zato MA: Surgical correction of high myopia in phakic eyes with Worst-Fechner myopia intraocular lenses. J Refract Surg 1997;13:268–281.

39 Pérez-Santonja JJ, Iradier MT, Benítez del Castillo JM, Serrano JM, Zato MA: Chronic subclinical inflammation in phakic eyes with intraocular lenses to correct myopia. J Cataract Refract Surg 1996;22:183–187.

40 Malecaze FJ, Hulin H, Bierer P, Fournié P, Grandjean H, Thalamas C, Guell JL: A randomized paired eye comparison of two techniques for treating moderately high myopia: LASIK and artisan phakic lens. Ophthalmology 2002;109:1622–1630.

41 Coullet J, Guëll J-L, Fournié P, Grandjean H, Gaytan J, Arné J-L, et al: Iris-supported phakic lenses (rigid vs foldable version) for treating moderately high myopia: randomized paired eye comparison. Am J Ophthalmol 2006;142:909–916.e2.

42 Baïkoff G, Bourgeon G, Jodai HJ, Fontaine A, Lellis FV, Trinquet L: Pigment dispersion and Artisan phakic intraocular lenses. J Cataract Refract Surg 2005;31:674–680.

43 Comaish IF, Lawless MA: Phakic intraocular lenses. Curr Opin Ophthalmol 2002;13:7–13.

44 Kohnen T, Mirshahi A, Hühren J, Kasper T, Baumaeister M: Complications of Phakic Intraocular Lenses. Principles and Practice. Thorofare, Slack, 2004, p 240.

45 Tahzib NG, Eggink FA, Frederik PM, Nuijts RM: Recurrent intraocular inflammation after implantation of the Artiflex phakic intraocular lens for the correction of high myopia. J Cataract Refract Surg 2006;32:1388–1391.

46 Güell JL, Morral M, Gris O, Gaytan J, Sisquella M, Manero F: Five-year follow-up of 399 phakic Artisan-Verisyse implantation for myopia, hyperopia, and/or astigmatism. Ophthalmology 2008;115:1002–1012.

47 Stulting RD, John ME, Maloney RK, Assil KK, Arrowsmith PN, Thompson VM, et al: Three-year results of Artisan/Verisyse phakic intraocular lens implantation. Results of the United States Food and Drug Administration clinical trial. Ophthalmology 2008;115:464–472.

48 Menezo JL, Cisneros AL, Rodriguez-Salvador V: Endothelial study of iris-claw phakic lenses: four year follow-up. J Cataract Refract Surg 1998;24:1039–1049.

49 Landesz M, Worst J, Van Rij G: Long-term results of correction of high myopia with an iris claw phakic intraocular lens. J Refract Surg 2000;16:310–316.

50 Budo C, Hessloehl JC, Izak M, Luyten GP, Menezo JL, Sener BA, et al: Multicenter study of the Artisan phakic intraocular lens. J Cataract Refract Surg 2000;26:1163–1171.

51 Pop M, Payette Y: Initial results of endothelial cell counts after Artisan lens for phakic eyes: an evaluation of the United States Food and Drug Administration Ophtec Study. Ophthalmology 2004;111:309–317.

52 Saxena R, Boekhoorn SS, Mulder PG, Noordzij B, van Rij G, Luyten GP: Long-term follow-up of endothelial cell change after Artisan phakic intraocular lens implantation. Ophthalmology 2008;115:608–613.

53 Coullet J, Gontran E, Fournié P, Arné JL, Malecaze F: Efficacité réfractive et tolérance de l'implant phaque myopique souple à fixation irienne Artiflex® dans la correction chirurgicale de la myopie forte: résultats à deux ans. J Fr Ophtalmol 2007;30:335–343.

54 Landesz M, van Rij G, Luyten G: Iris-claw phakic intraocular lens for high myopia. J Refract Surg 2001;17:634–640.

55 Maloney RK, Nguyen LH, John ME: Artisan phakic intraocular lens for myopia: short-term results of a prospective, multicenter study. Ophthalmology 2002;109:1631–1641.

56 Malecaze F, Hulin H, Bierer P: Iris-claw phakic (Artisan) lens to correct high myopia (in French). J Fr Ophtalmol 2002;23:879–883.

57 Menezo JL, Peris-Martínez C, Cisneros AL, Martínez-Costa R: Phakic intraocular lenses to correct high myopia: Adatomed, Staar, and Artisan. J Cataract Refract Surg 2004;30:33–44.

58 Alió JL, Mulet ME, Shalaby AM: Artisan phakic iris claw intraocular lens for high primary and secondary hyperopia. J Refract Surg 2002;18:697–707.

59 Saxena R, Landesz M, Noordzij B, Luyten GP: Three-year follow-up of the Artisan phakic intraocular lens for hypermetropia. Ophthalmology 2003;110:1391–1395.

60 Dick HB, Alió J, Bianchetti M, Budo C, et al: Toric phakic intraocular lens: European multicenter study. Ophthalmology 2003;110:150–162.

61 Güell JL, Vázquez M, Malecaze F, Manero F, Gris O, Velasco F, Hulin H, Pujol J: Artisan toric phakic intraocular lens for the correction of high astigmatism. Am J Ophthalmol 2003;136:442–447.

62 Zaldivar R, Davidorf JM, Oscherow S: Posterior chamber phakic intraocular lens for myopia of –8 to –19 diopters. J Refract Surg 1998;14:294–305.

63 Fyodorov SN, Zuyev VK, Aznabayev BM: Intraocular correction of high myopia with negative posterior chamber lens (in Russian). Oftalmokhirurgiia 1991;3:57–58.

64 Sanders DR, Martin RG, Brown DC, et al: Posterior chamber phakic intraocular lens for hyperopia. J Refract Surg 1999;15:309–315.

65 Gimbel HV, Ziémba SL: Management of myopic astigmatism with phakic intraocular lens implantation. J Cataract Refract Surg 2002;28:883–886.

66 Pallikaris IG, Kalyvianaki MI, Kymionis GD, Panagopoulou SI: Phakic refractive lens implantation in high myopic patients: one-year results. J Cataract Refract Surg 2004;30:1190–1197.

67 Arné JL, Hoang-Xuan T: Posterior chamber phakic IOL; in Azar DT (ed): IOLs in Cataract and Refractive Surgery. Philadelphia, WB Saunders, 2001, pp 267–272.

68 Asseto V, Benedetti S, Pesando P: Collamer intraocular contact lens to correct high myopia. J Cataract Refract Surg 1996;22:551–556.

69 Trindade F, Pereira F, Cronemberger S: Ultrasound biomicroscopic imaging of posterior chamber phakic intraocular lens. J Cataract Refract Surg 1998;14:497–503.

70 Jimenez-Alfaro I, Benitez del castillo JM, Garcia-Feijoo J, Gil de Bernabé JG, Serrano de la Iglesia JM: Safety of posterior chamber phakic intraocular lenses for the correction of high myopia; anterior segment changes after posterior chamber phakic intraocular lens implantation. Ophthalmology 2001;108:90–99.

71 Garcia Feijoo J, Jimenez Alfaro I, Cuina Sardina R, Mendez-Hernandez C, Benitez del Castillo JM, Garcia Sanchez J: Ultrasound biomicroscopy examination of posterior phakic lens position. Ophthalmology 2003;110:163–172.

72 Park SC, Kwun YK, Chung ES, Ahn K, Chung TY: Postoperative astigmatism and axis stability after implantation of the STAAR Toric Implantable Collamer Lens. J Refract Surg 2009;25:403–409.

73 Koivula A, Zetterström C: Phakic intraocular lens for the correction of hyperopia. J Cataract Refract Surg 2009;35:248–255.

74 Verde CM, Teus MA, Arranz-Marquez E, Cazorla RG: Medennium posterior chamber phakic refractive lens to correct high myopia. J Refract Surg 2007;23:900–904.

75 Sánchez-Galeana CA, Zadok D, Montes M, Cortés MA, Chayet AS: Refractory intraocular pressure increase after phakic posterior chamber intraocular lens implantation. Am J Ophthalmol 2002;134:121–123.

76 Arné JL, Lesueur LC: Phakic posterior chamber lenses for high myopia: functional and anatomical outcomes. J Cataract Refract Surg 2000;26:369–374.

77 Dejaco-Ruhswurm I, Scholz U, Pieh S, Hanselmayer G, Lackner B, Italon C, Ploner M, Skorpik C: Long-term endothelial changes in phakic eyes with posterior chamber intraocular lenses. J Cataract Refract Surg 2002;28:1589–1593.

78 Alfonso JF, Lisa C, Abdelhamid A, Montés-Micó R, Poo-López A, Ferrer-Blasco T: Posterior chamber phakic intraocular lenses after penetrating keratoplasty. J Cataract Refract Surg 2009;35:1166–1173.

79 Kamiya K, Shimizu K, Igarashi A, Hikita F, Komatsu M: Four-year follow-up of posterior chamber phakic intraocular lens implantation for moderate to high myopia. Arch Ophthalmol 2009;127:845–850.

80 Trindade F, Pereira F: Cataract formation after posterior chamber phakic intraocular lens implantation. J Cataract Refract Surg 1998;24:1661–1663.

81   Fink AM, Gore C, Rosen E: Cataract development after implantation of the Staar collamer posterior chamber phakic lens. J Cataract Refract Surg 1999;25:278–282.
82   Lackner B, Pieh S, Schmidinger G, Hanselmayer G, Dejaco-Ruhswurm I, Funovics MA, Skorpik C: Outcome after treatment of ametropia with implantable contact lenses. Ophthalmology 2003;110:2153–2161.
83   Chen LJ, Chang YJ, Kuo JC, Rajagopal R, Azar DT: Metaanalysis of cataract development after phakic intraocular lens surgery. J Cataract Refract Surg 2008;34:1181–1200.
84   ICL in Treatment of Myopia (ITM) Study Group: United States Food and Drug Administration clinical trial of the Implantable Collamer Lens (ICL) for moderate to high myopia. Ophthalmology 2003;110:255–266.
85   Kim DY, Reinstein DZ, Silverman RH, et al: Very high frequency ultrasound analysis of a new phakic posterior chamber intraocular lens in situ. Am J Ophthalmol 1998;125:725–729.
86   Hoyos JE, Dementiev DD, Cigales M, Hoyos-Chacón J, Hoffer KJ: Phakic refractive lens experience in Spain. J Cataract Refract Surg 2002;28:1939–1946.
87   Boxer Wachler BS, Scruggs RT, Yuen LH, Jalali S: Comparison of the Visian ICL and Verisyse phakic intraocular lenses for myopia from 6.00 to 20.00 diopters. J Refract Surg 2009;25:765–770.
88   Davidorf JM, Zaldivar R, Oscherow S: Posterior chamber phakic intraocular lens for hyperopia of +4 to +11 diopters. J Refract Surg 1998;14:306–311.

François Malecaze
Department of Ophthalmology
Purpan Hospital
FR–31024 Toulouse (France)
E-Mail malecaze.fr@chu-toulouse.fr

Güell JL (ed): Cataract. ESASO Course Series. Basel, Karger, 2013, vol 3, pp 100–115
DOI: 10.1159/000350912

Phakic Intraocular Lenses in Keratoconus

Jose L. Güell · Daniel Elies · Paula Verdaguer · Oscar Gris ·
Felicidad Manero · Merce Morral

Instituto Microcirugía Ocular, Universidad Autónoma de Barcelona, Barcelona, Spain

Abstract

There are several circumstances where phakic intraocular lenses (IOLs) might be considered in the management of the keratoconic patient, obviously only in the case of a stable refractive situation, sometimes difficult to be defined in this setting. Taking into account that the IOLs will only correct the sphere and the regular component of the astigmatism, sometimes they will be used in combination with other surgical strategies such as collagen crosslinking and/or intracorneal ring segments. In this chapter, we will evaluate the conceptual possible indications for them and review the published data as well as our own experience during these last 15 years.

Copyright © 2013 S. Karger AG, Basel

Keratoconus (KC), with a reported incidence of 1 per 2,000 in the general population, is a noninflammatory corneal disease that develops progressive thinning and anterior bulging of the cornea. Corneal ectasia frequently induces varied degrees of myopia and/or astigmatism [1]. In early stages, spectacles and contact lenses (CL) are the treatment of choice [2–4]. However, a considerable amount of patients with progressive KC have not only reduced visual acuity with spectacles due to irregular astigmatism [5, 6], but also reduced tolerance to CL [7–10].

Before the advent of modern refractive surgery techniques, penetrating keratoplasty or deep anterior lamellar keratoplasty was the treatment of choice when a patient with KC became CL intolerant or had poor best spectacle-corrected visual acuity.

This is still true in advanced stages of the disease, where severe thinning and/or corneal scarring occurs. Because refractive anisometropia and high postoperative astigmatism are common problems after penetrating keratoplasty, visual rehabilitation and return to binocular function may be slow [11–15]. Moreover, complications related to corneal transplant surgery itself, such as endophthalmitis or rejection episodes, should also be taken into account [16–21]. Therefore, in the early stages of KC when the central cornea remains clear, other options should be considered to avoid or delay keratoplasty.

With the exception of some anecdotal reports, corneal incisional (radial keratotomy, or arcuate keratotomy) and ablative refractive approaches such as photorefractive keratectomy (PRK) or LASIK are contraindicated in KC, as they increase the risk of progressive, irreversible corneal ectasia [22–25]. Available refractive procedures include intrastromal corneal ring segments (ICRS), and toric phakic intraocular lenses (TPIOLs). The main goal of these procedures is to provide enough best spectacle-corrected visual acuity, and sometimes uncorrected visual acuity, to postpone the need for a corneal transplantation.

Intracorneal rings provide structural reinforcement of the cornea, and reshape and center cornea's optical zone, improving topographic abnormalities (irregular astigmatism), quality of vision and visual acuity [26–29]. Intracorneal rings act as spacing elements that shorten the arc of the length of the anterior corneal surface and flatten the central cornea, which reduces the myopic spherical equivalent [30–32]. However, they only correct a limited range of myopia, and high refractive errors may remain. Residual refractive errors may be corrected with spectacles or soft or hard CL [33]. TPIOLs have also been implanted after ICRS [34–36].

In the same way [37, 38] that toric pseudophakic IOLs have been used when cataract is present, PIOLs have been used to correct moderate and high myopia, hyperopia and/or astigmatism. There are also a few reports on their use in patients with KC [39–41]. The implantation of PIOLs has been reported to be a stable, predictable and safe refractive procedure [42–52].

Some authors proposed UVA irradiation-induced corneal collagen crosslinking (CXL) as a first step to stop the progression of KC [53–57]. Also, although the role of ICRS in stopping the progression of KC is still controversial, some authors have implanted first the rings and then the TPIOL with a similar goal.

Several clinical trials have shown the efficacy of corneal CXL in stopping the progression of KC [58]. CXL performed before or after ICRS implantation in keratoconic eyes provided better results, as evidenced by greater reductions in manifest cylinder and keratometry readings. A simple additive effect of both procedures in flattening the central cornea and greater local rigidity across the ICRS segment may account for this synergistic effect [59, 60].

Topography-guided surface ablations combined with CXL have also been proposed [57, 61–64].

However, given the evidence available to date, corneal ablation procedures should be performed with caution, especially in higher corrections, because there is an increased risk for triggering progressive irreversible corneal ectasia when corneal laser ablations are performed in keratoconic eyes [22–25].

Before the advent of CXL, correcting refractive errors with PIOLs in cases of progressive KC was not advisable because the refractive correction and uncorrected distance visual acuity (UDVA) achieved would not be maintained over the long term. Izquierdo et al. [65] reported that combined CXL and iris claw Artiflex PIOL (Ophtec BV) implantation was safe and effective in 11 eyes with grade I–II progressive KC and less than –2.50 dpt of astigmatism after 12 months.

Later on, Güell et al. [66] published their experience with the Toric Artiflex, and some other reports have been presented worldwide (fig. 1).

Visual rehabilitation of KC should always involve (1) stabilization of the cone if required (some keratoconic eyes are already stable at the time of diagnosis); (2) correction, if significant, of the irregular component (irregular astigmatism), and (3) correction of regular refractive errors either by optical or surgical means (fig. 2). Stabilization of the cone is essential in order to obtain a long-lasting refractive correction that provides functional vision. When functional vision cannot be achieved by any of the available surgical options, which is generally due to high levels of irregular astigmatism, the remaining viable option is a corneal graft (fig. 3).

Corneal Collagen Crosslinking Combined with Other Corneal Refractive Surgery Techniques

In cases with clinically significant irregular astigmatism, we may consider intracorneal ring implantation with the aim to regularize the anterior corneal surface and, thus, decrease anterior distortion and improve corrected distance visual acuity (CDVA) [26–29, 32, 67–69] (fig. 4, 5).

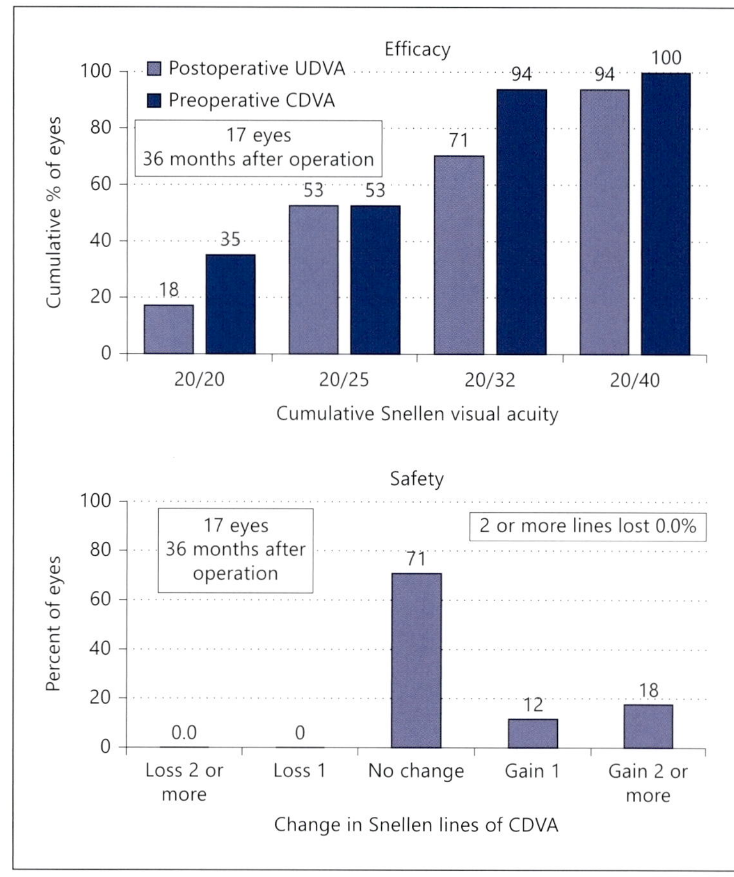

Fig. 1a. VA data in this study group.

In a considerable number of cases, such irregular astigmatism compensation, together with the regular spherocylindrical component, is usually properly achieved by the adaptation of some of the different styles of rigid gas-permeable CL (RGPCL). CXL performed before or after intracorneal ring implantation in keratoconic eyes has shown a synergistic effect, demonstrated by greater reductions in manifest cylinder and keratometry readings [59, 60]. The order of implementation of both procedures providing the best outcomes is still under debate. TPIOLs may also be used in combination with ICRS to refine residual refractive errors [60] (fig. 6, 7).

Topography-guided surface ablations combined with CXL have also been proposed [57, 61,

63, 64, 70]. However, with the evidence available to the date, corneal ablation procedures should be taken with caution, especially in higher corrections, as there is a demonstrated increased risk of triggering progressive, irreversible corneal ectasia when corneal ablations are performed in keratoconic eyes [22–25].

Corneal Collagen Crosslinking Combined with Phakic Intraocular Lenses

PIOLs have been proven effective and safe for the correction of a wide range of refractive errors. Outcomes of PIOL implantation in non-progressive, keratoconic eyes are comparable to non-

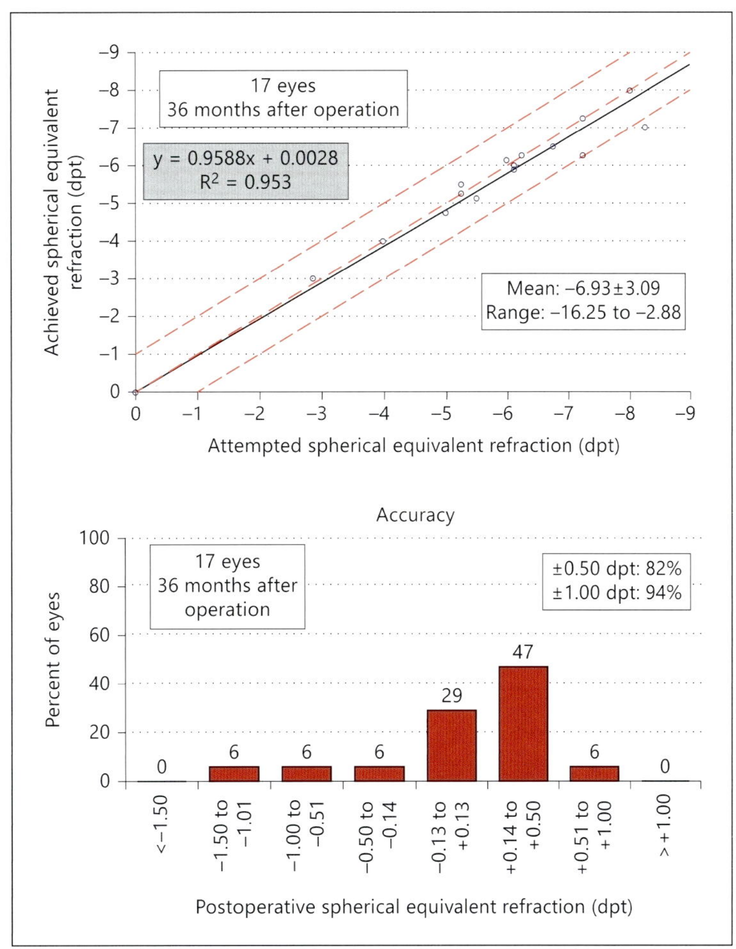

Fig. 1b. SE results in this study group.

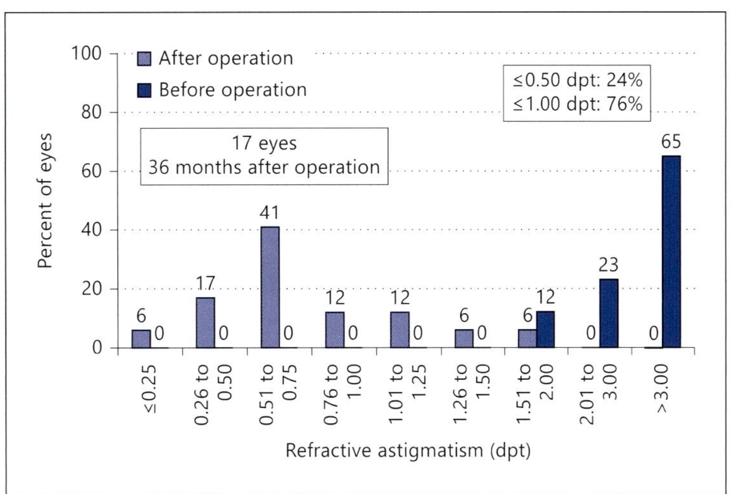

Fig. 1c. Refractive astigmatism results in this study group.

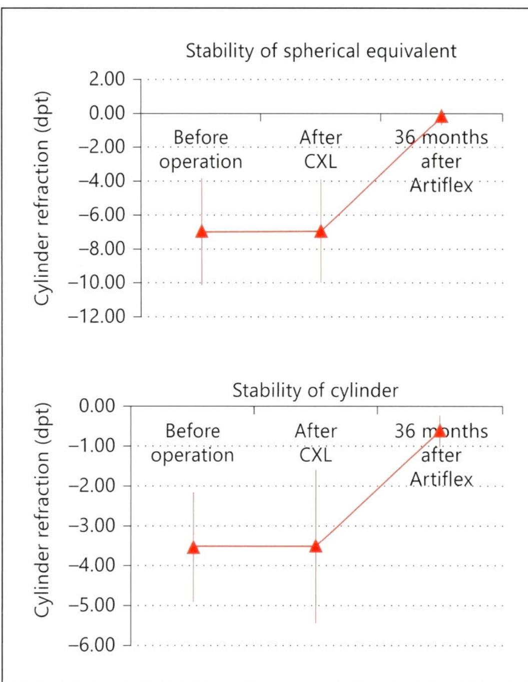

Fig. 1d. First 3 years mean and SD SE and astigmatism postoperative stability results in the same study.

keratoconic eyes in terms of efficacy, safety, and stability of refractive results [42, 44, 50, 71–77]. Although implantable collamer lenses (Staar Surgical, Monrovia, Calif., USA) have been proposed as a valid alternative for the correction of the stable myopic astigmatism in patients with KC [78–80], we believe that the iris claw PIOL (either toric or spherical, depending on the case) is a better option for these patients, especially when correcting astigmatism. The unique enclavation system prevents any potential rotation of the lens, which would result in the loss of the refractive correction effect [81–83]. However, as toric iris claw style PIOLs are not commercially available in the US yet, full correction of the astigmatism with spherical PIOLs is limited.

Clinical data on the combination of CXL and PIOLs for the correction of refractive errors in patients with KC are scarce [65, 66, 84]. Both an-

terior chamber, iris claw and posterior chamber PIOLs have been used, but there is no report on angle-supported PIOLs yet. As a general rule, CXL is performed first to stabilize the cone, followed by PIOL implantation once refractive and topographic stability is documented.

Indications and Contraindications of Collagen Crosslinking and Phakic Intraocular Lenses

The protocol for the treatment of KC used in our institution (the Instituto de Microcirugia Ocular, Barcelona, Spain) is summarized in figure 2 [66]. The combination of CXL and PIOL implantation is indicated in patients (usually of young age) with documented progressive KC, CL intolerant or who seek refractive surgery and present moderate to high refractive errors, including myopia, hyperopia and/or astigmatism, and no clinically significant irregular astigmatism.

Patients with clinically significant irregular astigmatism or CDVA <20/50 are generally excluded. Irregular astigmatism is deemed clinically significant when the CDVA achieved with spectacles is at least one line worse than CDVA measured with RGPCL. Other standard inclusion criteria are: clear cornea; corneal thinnest point >450 μm as measured by ultrasound (US) pachymetry; central anterior chamber depth >3.0 mm, measured from the corneal endothelium to the anterior surface of the crystalline lens; cECC >2,300 cells/mm^2; normal iris morphology and pupil function; light mesopic pupil size <4.5 mm; absence of other ocular pathology or systemic disease which may alter the healing response of both procedures.

Diagnosis of KC is based on clinical and topographic data. Generally speaking, at least four of the following topographic signs should be present: (1) an irregular keratometric map suggesting irregular astigmatism (inferior steepening, asymmetric bow tie, or skewed radial axes); (2) increased anterior best fit sphere; (3) posterior best fit sphere >45 μm; (4) inferior and/or nasal-temporal decentration of

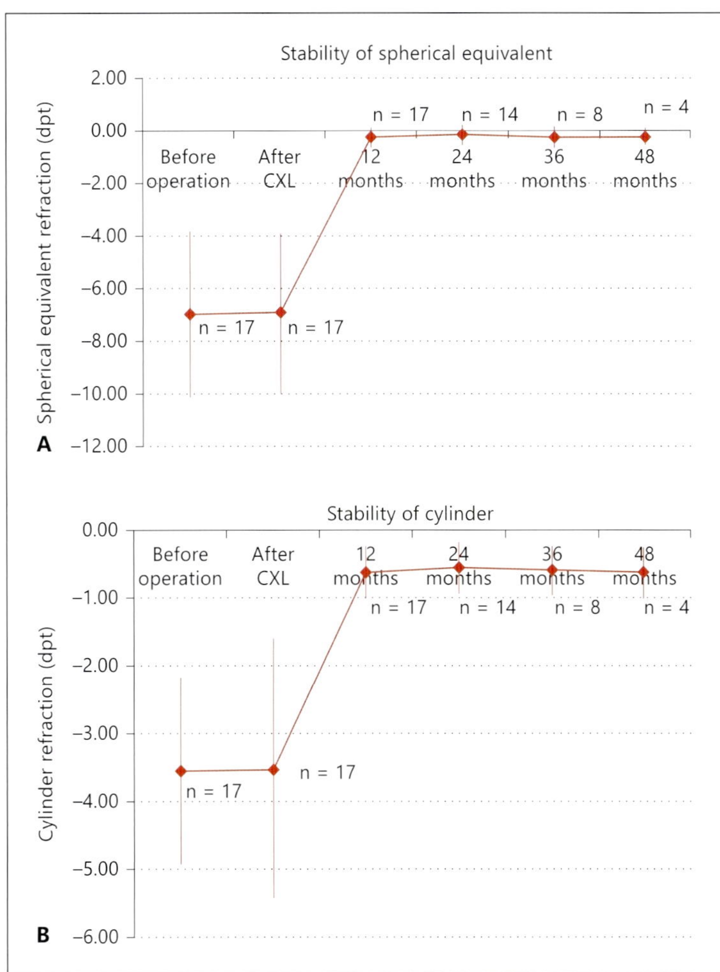

Fig. 1e. First 4 years SE and astigmatism postoperative stability results in the same study.

the maximum point of anterior and/or posterior corneal elevation; (5) coincidences of apices and corneal thinnest point; (6) asymmetry of inferior-superior and/or nasal-temporal pachymetry >50 μm; (7) difference between central and peripheral pachymetry >100 μm at any point.

Progression of KC is diagnosed when one or more of the following are present: refractive shift (especially changes in cylinder magnitude and/or axis) of more than 0.75 dpt; increase on corneal SimK >1 dpt, and/or decrease in ultrasound corneal pachymetry >25 μm demonstrated in at least two consecutive examinations 6–12 months apart.

Surgical Technique

Written informed consent to perform the surgical procedure is obtained from all patients before surgery in accordance with the Declaration of Helsinki, and they are asked to give their consent to use their data for research. All patients are warned of the benefits and potential risks of both surgeries, and the potential progression of KC and subsequent change in their refractive error despite CXL.

Our experience is based on the use of iris claw PIOLs. We consider this type of PIOLs presents

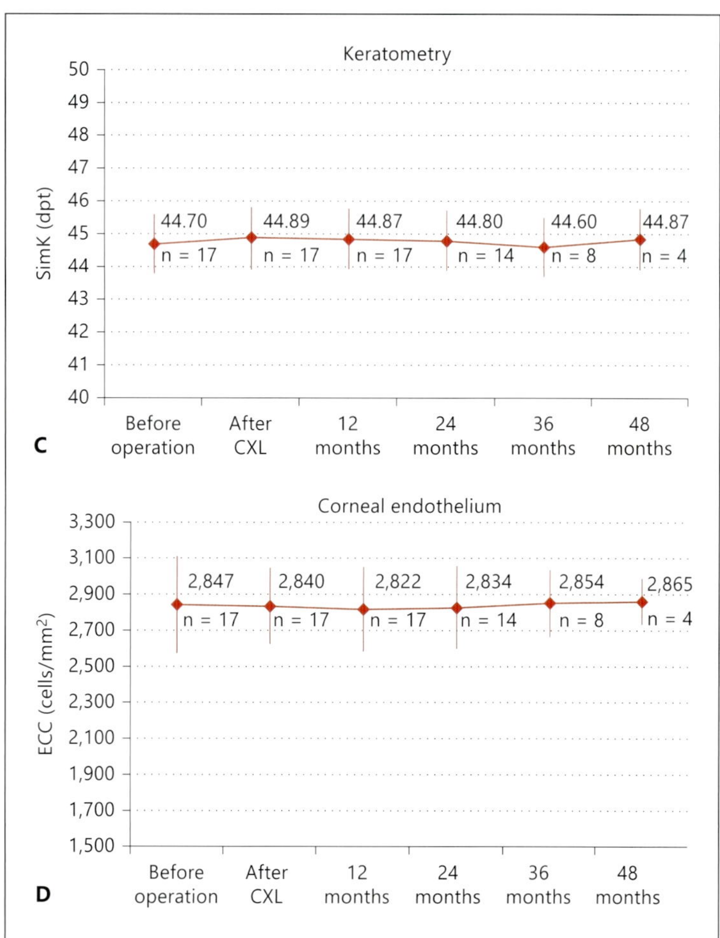

Fig. 1e. Postoperative evolution of mean topographic keratometry and central endothelial cell count in the same study.

several advantages over other designs, which include: (1) preservation of anterior chamber angle structures; (2) greater distance to the endothelium than angle-supported PIOLs (decreased risk of endothelial damage); (3) greater distance to the crystalline lens than posterior chamber PIOLs (decreased risk of cataract formation); (4) no contact with the pigmentary epithelium of the iris (decreased risk of future pigmentary glaucoma); (5) adequate centration over the pupil even if off center; (6) fixation system provides stability of astigmatic corrections [42, 71, 73].

CXL is performed first, and Toric Artiflex implantation is performed once the stability of manifest refraction and topography are achieved, usually between 3 and 6 months after CXL. CXL is performed using the standard technique described as in the Dresden protocol.

Toric Phakic Iris Claw Artiflex/Artisan Implantation after Collagen Crosslinking

Once stability is confirmed by two consecutive manifest refraction and topography measurements separated by at least one month, Artiflex/Artisan PIOL implantation is performed. As KC generally presents with astigmatism, the toric

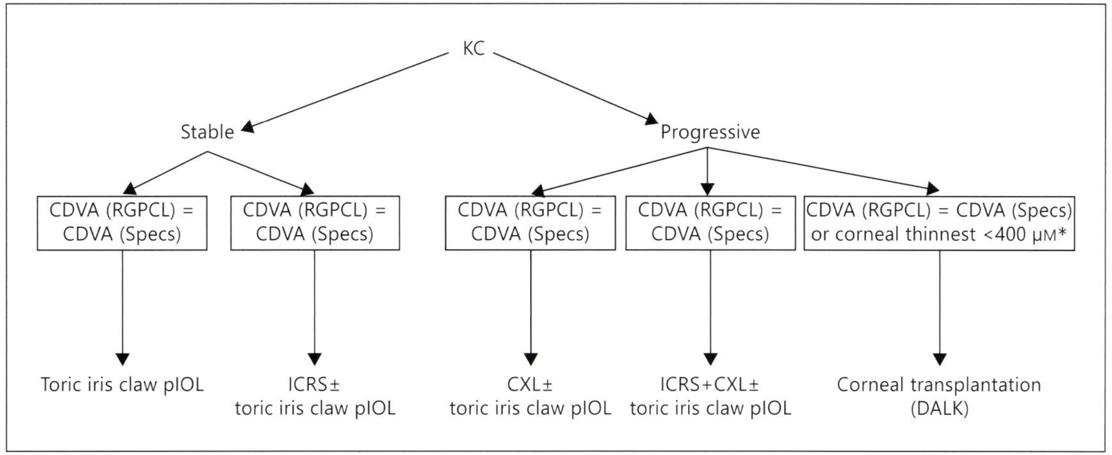

Fig. 2. Protocol for the management of KC in CL-intolerant patients. Decisions are made considering the stability of the cone and vision. CXL is performed only in cases of proven progressive KC. In cases with no clinically significant irregular astigmatism (i.e. when the CDVA with RGPCL is the same as spectacle-corrected distance visual acuity), a toric iris claw pIOL implantation might be the technique of choice to correct myopic astigmatism. In the presence of significant irregular astigmatism, ICRS are implanted first to regularize corneal topography (some cases could be managed with topography-guided PRK and CXL). Phakic IOLs might also be used to correct residual myopic astigmatism. In progressive keratoconic eyes, CXL is performed first to stop the progression of the cone as long as CDVA is 20/50 or better and corneal pachymetry at the thinnest point is at least 400 mm. Corneal transplantation is the procedure of choice in cases of advanced KC with corneal scarring and poor vision. Specs = Spectacles. Asterisk indicates that hyposmotic riboflavin solution may be used if corneal thinnest point is <400 μm.

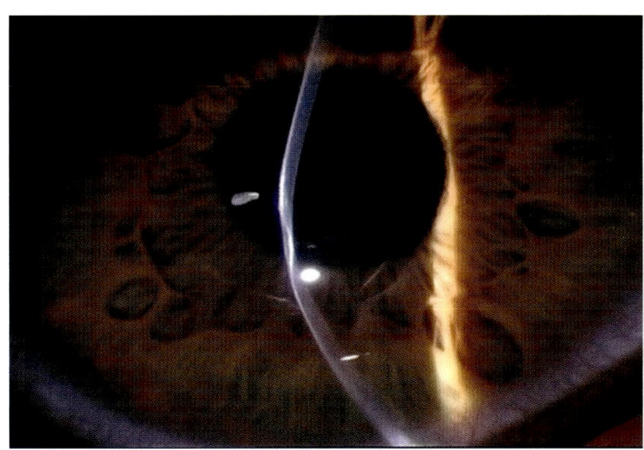

Fig. 3. Primary KC. In some posthydrops situations and when keratoplasty is indicated, deep anterior lamellar techniques might not be considered because of the high risk of peroperative perforation and the possible residual central opacity.

model is the most frequently used (surgical technique, fig. 8).

The Toric Artiflex PIOL (Ophtec, Groningen, the Netherlands) consists of a flexible optical part made of ultraviolet-absorbing silicone and two rigid haptics made of Perspex CQ UV polymethyl methacrylate (PMMA). The lens is currently available from –2.0 to –14.5 dpt, with a torus from –1 to –5 dpt. If the preoperative astigmatism is higher than –5 dpt, the PMMA model (Toric Artisan PIOL), which is available from +12 to –23.5 dpt, with a cylinder from –1.0 to –7.0 dpt, is used. The lens power is calculated using the modified Van der Heijde formula, which uses the mean corneal curvature, adjusted ACD, and the manifest refraction at the spectacle plane at 12 mm [85].

The 180° axis is marked with the use of a needle on the ophthalmometer with the patient in a

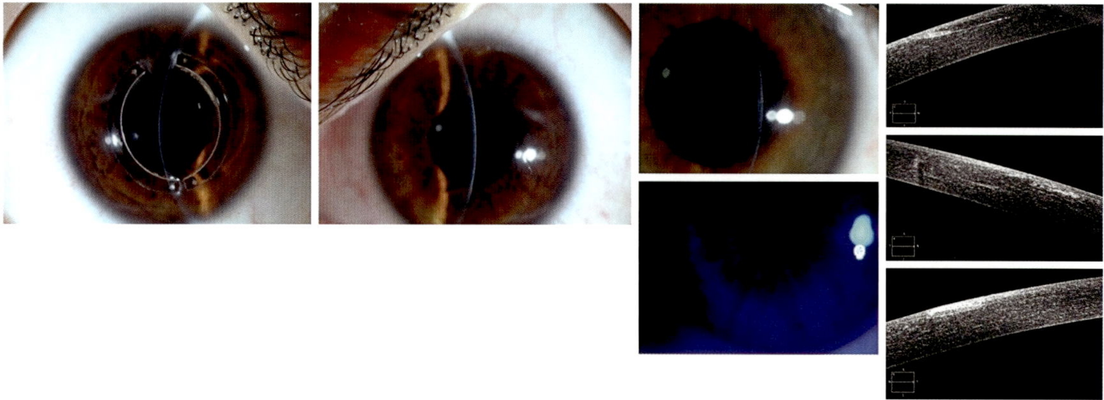

Fig. 4. Patient with secondary corneal ectasia some years after LASIK. We performed CXL in both eyes to stabilize the situation and implanted Intacts on the right eye to improve the residual irregular astigmatism. On the slit lamp images and high-definition OCT (Cirrus), it is easy to observe the old LASIK lenticule.

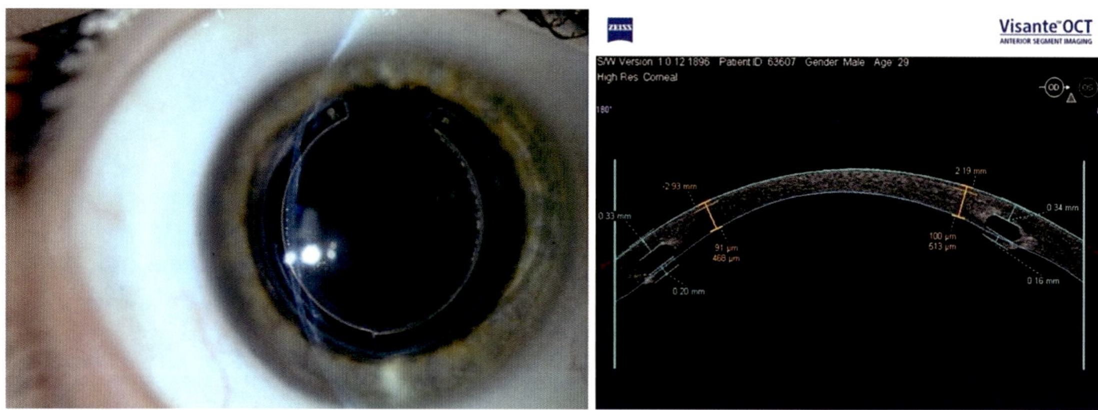

Fig. 5. This is one of the most common Intacts positions when correcting KC-associated corneal irregular astigmatism in our practice: two segments embracing the inferior part of the cone.

seated position to avoid implantation errors due to cyclotorsion and/or positional changes (a relevant anatomic landmark at the limbus is also frequently used). When the foldable model is implanted, topical anesthesia is used, and a 3.2-mm, vascular, one-plane, posterior cornea incision is performed. When the PMMA model is used, peri- or retrobulbar anesthesia is injected, and a two-plane 5.2-mm posterior corneal

incision is performed. The center of the pupil is marked on the cornea at the beginning of the surgery, to allow correct centration of the PIOL over the pupil. Acetylcholine (Myochol) is injected in the anterior chamber at the beginning of the procedure. Preoperative drops of pilocarpine 1% are not generally used in order not to change the physiological position of the pupil before the surgery. After the anterior chamber is

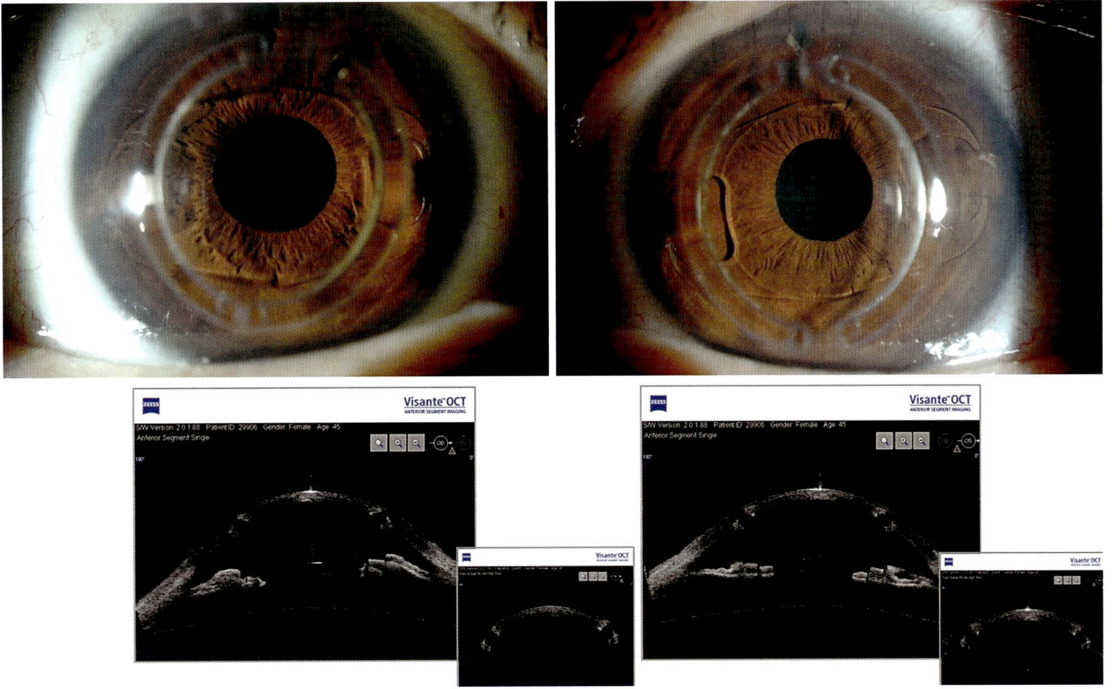

Fig. 6. Two examples of where we combined the use of CXL to stabilize the cone, Intacts ICRS to improve irregular astigmatism (SK in the second case, with a smaller optical zone and section shape, in order to increase its effect) and a TPIOL (Artisan-Artiflex) to correct the final residual ammetropia.

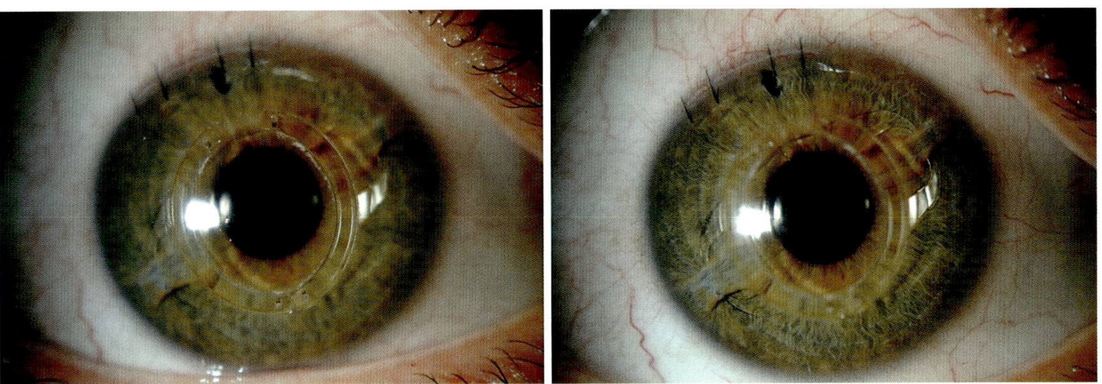

Fig. 7. The same combination, ICRS and toric artisan in a stable stage III keratoconic patient.

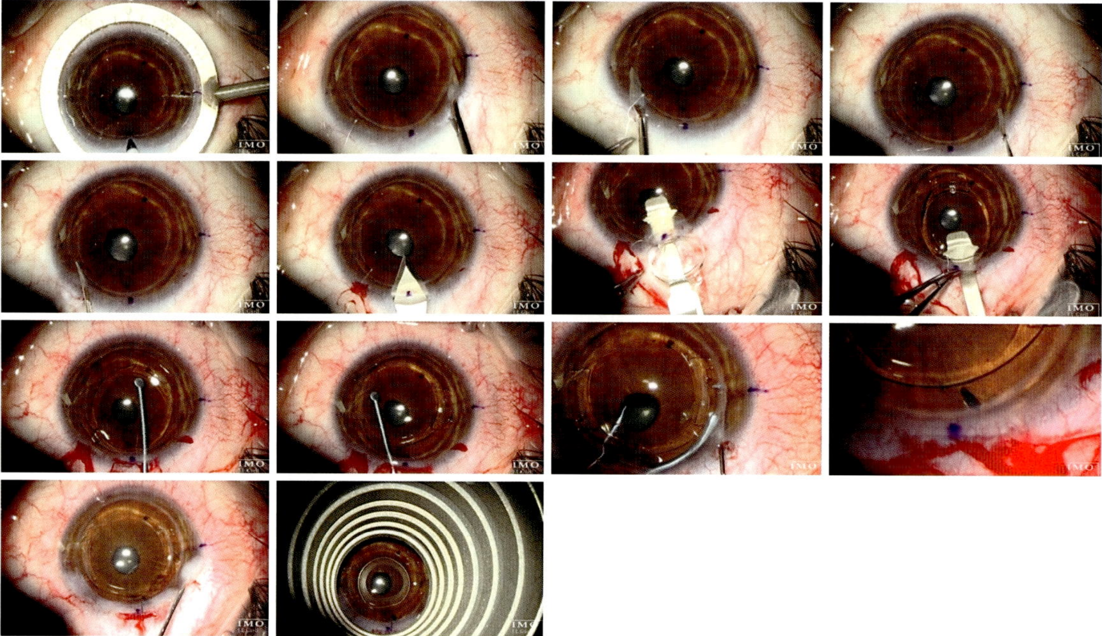

Fig. 8. Series of surgical steps when implanting a toric phakic Artiflex to correct the residual ammetropia after deep anterior keratoplasty in a CL-intolerant patient with advanced KC. Preoperative proper axis alignment is mandatory. It is also extremely important performing peripheral iridectomy and evaluating an adequate suture tension at the end of the surgery.

filled with a cohesive viscoelastic, the IOL is introduced with a specially designed spatula, and rotated up to the desired orientation of implantation. Then, the lens is fixed with the use of an enclavation needle. Both fixation of the iris claws and proper centration of the PIOL over the pupil are checked. A peripheral iridectomy with 25-gauge vitreoretinal forceps and scissors is performed to prevent pupillary block glaucoma. Alternatively, intraoperative iridectomy with a vitrectome or 2 small preoperative iridotomies with a neodymium:YAG laser can also be used. The 3.2-mm incision is usually watertight, but we prefer to place a 10-0 nylon interrupted suture. The 5.2-mm incision (for the PMMA model) is closed with 5 interrupted 10-0 nylon sutures, which are gradually taken out, starting 6 weeks postoperatively, to minimize surgery-induced astigmatism.

Results

In progressive KC, PIOL implantation alone would not provide stable refractive results in the mid- and long-term. Therefore, CXL is performed first to stop the progression of the cone (fig. 9, 10). Only 2 small case series have reported the results of the combination of CXL and PIOL implantation. In March 2012, we published the clinical and refractive data of 17 eyes of 9 patients with progressive KC and myopic astigmatism who consequently underwent CXL combined with iris claw toric Artisan/Artiflex PIOL implantation from November 2006 to July 2009 [66] (fig. 1). Previously, Izquierdo et al. [65] had published the results of 11 eyes that underwent CXL combined with spherical Artiflex PIOL implantation. The only report on CXL and posterior chamber PIOL is a case report published by Kymionis

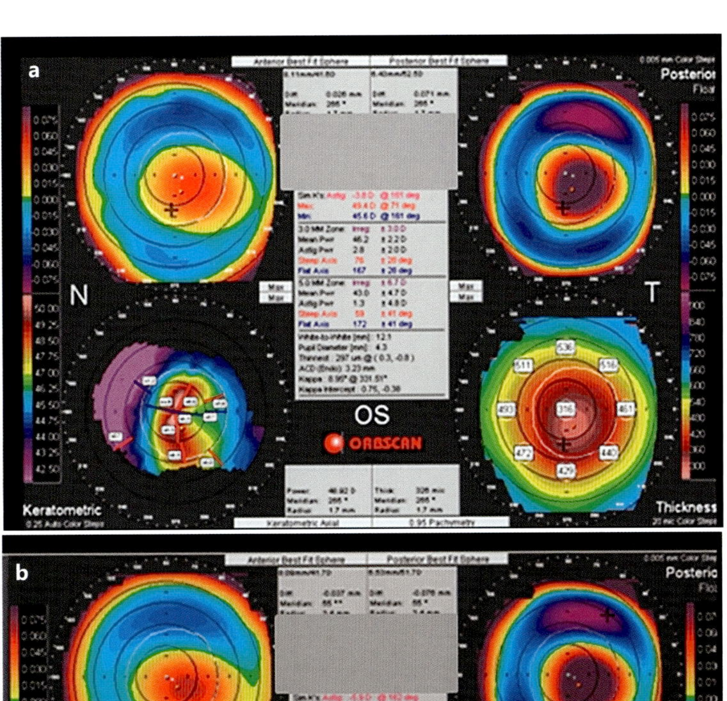

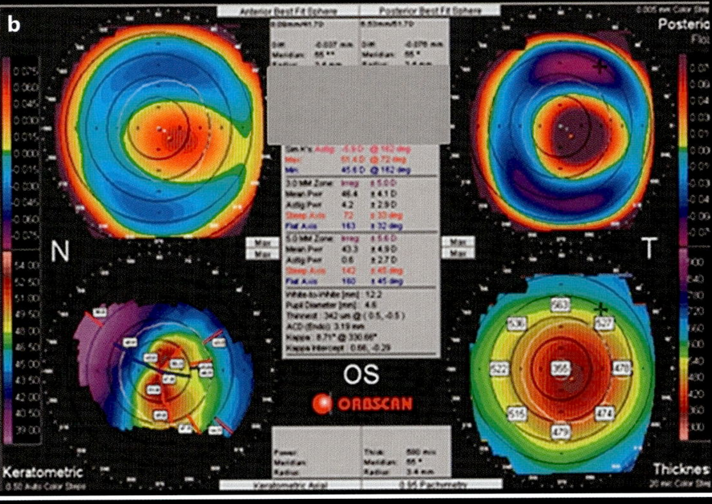

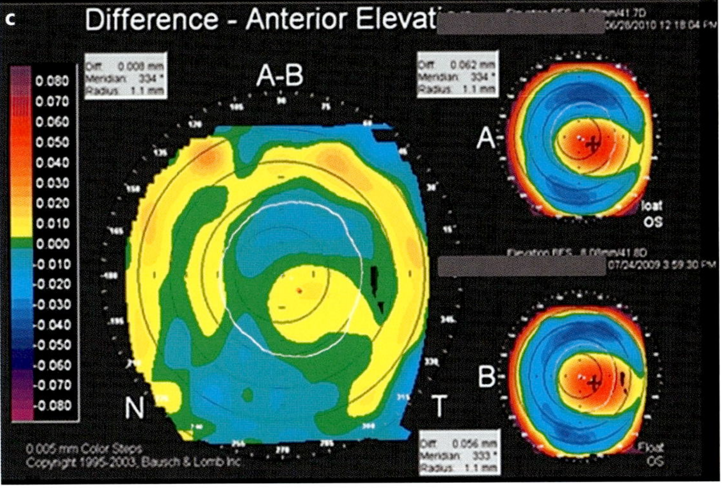

Fig. 9. Orbscan topographies of a patient with progressive KC. **a** Precorneal CXL. **b** 5 months after CXL. **c** Anterior elevation difference map before vs. after CXL. Stability of the KC can be observed (from the post CXL period to the end of the follow up).

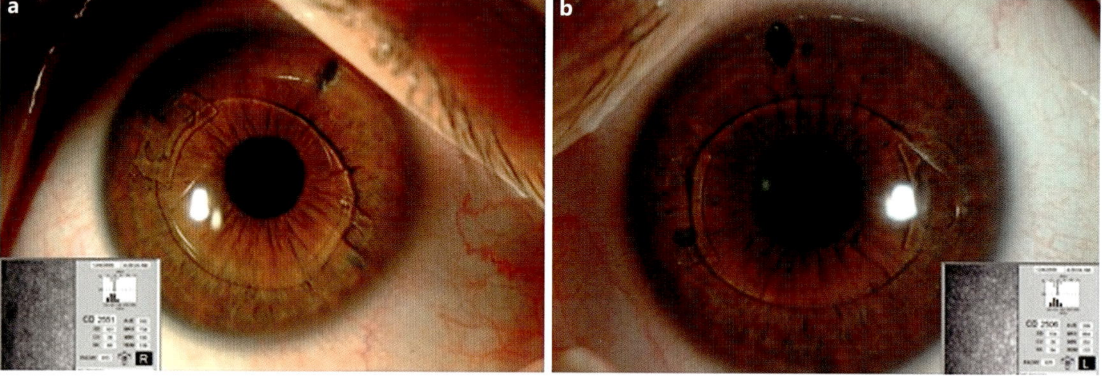

Fig. 10. Postoperative clinical photograph and central ECC of the right eye (OD; **a**) and left eye (OS; **b**) of a 21-year-old male with KC who underwent corneal CXL and Toric Artiflex implantation. Preoperative CDVA was 20/40 OD with 25° –3.00 to –4.50, and 20/20 OS with 100° –3.50 to –4.00. Fourteen months after Toric Artiflex PIOL implantation, OD presented UDVA and CDVA of 20/30 OD with 30° –0.25, and OS UDVA 20/25, and CDVA 20/20 with 105° –1.00 to +0.50.

et al. [84], who performed posterior chamber toric implantable collamer lens (Visian ICL; STAAR Surgical) implantation 12 months after corneal CXL with riboflavin and UVA on a 29-year-old woman with KC, with excellent visual and refractive results. Three months postoperatively, UDVA improved from counting fingers to 20/40 and CDVA improved from 20/100 to 20/30.

Izquierdo et al. [65] suggested a minimal interval between CXL and Artiflex PIOL implantation of 6 months to consider the changes produced by the CXL procedure on refractive errors and keratometric values, which affect the calculation of the PIOL power. Their series of 11 eyes demonstrated a reduction in mean maximum keratometry of 1.27 dpt 6 months after CXL, and 2.14 dpt 6 months after spherical non-Toric Artiflex PIOL implantation (12 months after CXL) [65]. In our study, the median interval between CXL and PIOL implantation was 3.9 ± 0.7 months, with a maximum of 5 months. As we did not observe any decrease in spherical equivalent or keratometry in any of our patients, and as we did not find any significant changes in mean K or K_{max} throughout the follow-up either, a longer interval between the two procedures would not have changed the final outcome.

Nevertheless, there is still no consensus on the appropriate interval between CXL and PIOL implantation. Some investigators have observed a temporary reduction in CDVA after CXL. If this occurs, we recommend delaying the implantation surgery until CDVA has reached at least preoperative values.

With 94% of the eyes within 0.5 dpt of attempted spherical equivalent correction, and 76% of the eyes within 1 dpt of attempted cylinder correction, our study showed comparable results to iris claw PIOLs used in non-keratoconic eyes [42, 44, 71–75]. No significant changes in spherical equivalent and cylinder, or in minimum, maximum and mean keratometry (neither steepening nor flattening) were observed throughout the follow-up period (p > 0.05), which demonstrates the stabilizing effect of CXL.

We did not observe any serious intraoperative or postoperative complications. Izquierdo et al. [65] reported transient, mild haze in 2/11 (18%) eyes. Both eyes of one of our patients required longer topical steroid treatment because of a tendency to accumulate giant and pigmentary cells on the optic surface of the Artiflex PIOL, which completely cleared after 4 weeks of treatment with topical steroids and mydriatic drops.

Safety data compare favorably with non-keratoconic eyes with none of the eyes losing any line of CDVA. Similar to the European Multicenter Study of the Artisan® PIOL [86], the US FDA Ophtec Study [45], and our 5-year follow-up of 399 eyes [42], we did not find any significant loss of endothelial cell density throughout the follow-up period. These results suggest that the combination of CXL and Toric Artiflex does not result in any additional loss. Nonetheless, ECC should be monitored at yearly intervals in all patients as long-term studies have reported a significant decrease in endothelial cell counts (ECCs) of about 9% at 5 and 10 years [75, 87, 88].

It should be remembered that:

- Still today, most KC patients are being managed by nonsurgical means (spectacles and CL).
- As KC is a progressive disease, its stability should be confirmed before undertaking any refractive surgery procedure.
- CXL is the only treatment available with demonstrated efficacy in stopping the progression of KC.
- Pseudophakic IOL and PIOL implantation has shown excellent efficacy and safety in correcting moderate to high regular refractive errors in both keratoconic and non-keratoconic eyes.
- CXL combined with PIOL implantation is indicated in progressive KC with CL intolerance, good CDVA, and absence of irregular astigmatism and/or corneal opacities.
- After CXL, in cases with clinically significant irregular astigmatism, visual rehabilitation and good CDVA can be achieved with special RGPCL, which provide good CDVA in most cases. If CDVA is not good enough with RGPCL or the patient is intolerant to them, intracorneal rings may be considered to regularize the anterior corneal surface and, thus, decrease irregular astigmatism and improve CDVA (topography-guided PRK and CXL might also be considered).

In conclusion, CXL combined with PIOL implantation constitutes a promising therapeutic approach for progressive KC with moderate to high refractive errors, regular astigmatism and good CDVA. However, longer follow-up clinical data from prospective randomized clinical trials are needed to confirm its effectiveness and safety.

References

1 Rabinowitz YS: Keratoconus. Surv Ophthalmol 1998;42:297–319.
2 Riddle HK, Parker DA, Price FW: Management of postkeratoplasty astigmatism. Curr Opin Ophthalmol 1998;9:15–28.
3 Chastang PJ, Borderie VM, Carvajal-Gonzalez S, et al: Prediction of spectacle-corrected visual acuity using videokeratography. J Refract Surg 1999;15:572–579.
4 Speaker MG, Cohen EJ, Edelhauser HF, et al: Effect of gas-permeable contact lenses on the endothelium of corneal transplants. Arch Ophthalmol 1991;109:1703–1706.
5 Busin M, Arffa RC, Zambiachi L, et al: Effect of hinged lamellar keratotomy on postkeratoplasty eyes. Ophthalmology 2001;108:1845–1854, discussion 1851–1852.
6 Vaipayee RB, Sharma N, Sinha R, et al: Laser in situ keratomileusis after penetrating keratoplasty. Surv Ophthalmol 2003;48:503–514.
7 Lim N, Vogt U: Characteristics and functional outcomes of 130 patients with keratoconus attending specialist contact lens clinic. Eye 2002;16:54–59.
8 Geerards AJ, Vreugdebhil W, Khazen A: Incidence of rigid gas-permeable contact lens wear after keratoplasty for keratoconus. Eye Contact Lens 2006;32:207–210.
9 España EM, Tseng SC: Analysis of contact lens intolerance by exploring neuroanatomic integration of ocular surface defense. Cont Lens Anterior Eye 2003;26:131–137.
10 Glasson MJ, Stapleton F, Keav L, et al: Invest Ophthalmol Vis Sci 2003;44:5116–5124.
11 Thompson RW Jr, Price MO, Bowers PJ, Price FW: Long-term graft survival after penetrating keratoplasty. Ophthalmology 2003;110:1396–1402.
12 Lim L, Pseudovs K, Coster DJ: Penetrating keratoplasty for keratoconus: visual outcome and success. Ophthalmology 2000;107:1125–1131.
13 Brooks SF, Johnson D, Fischer N: Anisometropia and binocularity. Ophthalmology 1996;103:1139–1143.
14 Perlman EM: An analysis and interpretation of refractive errors after penetrating keratoplasty. Ophthalmolgy 1981;88:39–45.
15 Perl T, Charlton KH, Binder PS: Disparate diameter grafting. Astigmatism, intraocular pressure, and visual acuity. Ophthalmology 1981;88:774–781.

16 Kruse FE, Cursifien C: Surgery of the cornea: corneal, limbal stem cell and amniotic membrane transplantation. Dev Ophthalmol 2008;41:159–170.

17 Frost NA, Wu J, Lai TF, Coster DJ: A review of randomized controlled trials of penetrating keratoplasty techniques. Ophthalmology 2006;113:942–949.

18 Chang DH, Hardten DR: Refractive surgery after corneal transplantation. Curr Opin Ophthalmol 2005;16:251–255.

19 Taban M, Behrens A, Newcomb RL, et al: Incidence of acute endophthalmitis following penetrating keratoplasty: a systematic review. Arch Ophthalmol 2005;123:605–609.

20 Patel HY, Omonde S, Brookes NH, et al: The indications and outcome of paediatric corneal transplantation in New Zealand: 1991–2003. Br J Ophthalmol 2005; 89:404–408.

21 Panda A, Vanathi M, Kumar A, et al: Corneal graft rejection. Surv Ophthalmol 2007;52:375–396.

22 Randleman JB, Woodward M, Lynn MJ, Stulting RD: Risk assessment for ectasia after corneal refractive surgery. Ophthalmology 2008;115:37–50.

23 Randleman JB, Russell B, Ward MA, et al: Risk factors and prognosis for corneal ectasia after LASIK. Ophthalmology 2003;110:267–275.

24 Randleman JB, Trattler WB, Stulting RD: Validation of the Ectasia Risk Score System for preoperative laser in situ keratomileusis screening. Am J Ophthalmol 2008;145:813–818.

25 Binder PS: Analysis of actasia after laser in situ keratomileusis: risk factors. J Cataract Refrac Surg 2007;33:1530–1538.

26 Colin J: European clinical evaluation: use of Intacts for the treatment of keratoconus. J Cataract Refract Surg 2006;32: 747–755.

27 Colin J, Cochener B, Savary G, Malet F: Correcting keratoconus with intracorneal rings. J Cataract Refract Surg 2000; 26:1117–1122.

28 Colin J, Cochener B, Savary G, et al: INTACTS inserts for treating keratoconus; one year results. Ophthalmology 2001; 108:1409–1414.

29 Siganos D, Ferrara F, Chatzinikolas K, et al: Ferrara intrastromal corneal rings for the correction of keratoconus. J Cataract Refract Surg 2002;28:1947–1951.

30 Holmes-Higgin DK, Burris TE: Corneal surface topography and associated visual performance with Intacts for myopia: phase III clinical trials results. The Intacts Study Group. Ophthalmology 2000;107:2061–2071.

31 Schanzlin DJ, Asbell PA, Burris DS: The Intrastromal corneal ring segments: phase II results for the correction of myopia. Ophthalmology 1997;104:1067–1078.

32 Pokroy R, Levinger S: Intacts adjustment surgery for keratoconus. J Cataract Refract Surg 2006;32:986–992.

33 Ucakhan OO, Kanpolat A, Ozdemir O: Contact lens fitting for keratoconus after Intacts placement. Eye Contact Lens 2006;32:75–77.

34 Kamburoglu G, Etan A, Bahadir M: Implantation of Artisan toric phakic intraocular lens following Intacts in a patient with keratoconus. J Cataract Refract Surg 2007;33:528–530.

35 Colin J, Velou S: Implantation of Intacs and a refractive intraocular lens to correct keratoconus. J Cataract Refract Surg 2003;29:832–834.

36 Coskinseven E, Onder M, Kymionis GD, et al: Combined Intacts and posterior chamber toric implantable collamer lens implantation for keratoconic patients with extreme myopia. Am J Ophthalmol 2007;144:387–389.

37 Visser N, Gast ST JM, Bauer NJC, Nuijts RMMA: Cataract surgery with toric intraocular lens implantation in keratoconus: a case report. Cornea 2011;30:720–723.

38 Sauder G, Jonas JB: Treatment of keratoconus by Toric foldable intraocular lenses. Eur J Ophthalmol 2003;13:577–579.

39 Moshirfar M, Gregoire FJ, Mirzaian G, et al: Use of Verisyse iris-supported phakic intraocular lens for myopia in keratoconic patients. J Cataract Refract Surg 2006;32:1227–1232.

40 Leccisotti A, Fields SV: Angle-supported phakic intraocular lenses in eyes with keratoconus and myopia. J Cataract Refract Surg 2003;29:1530–1536.

41 Budo C, Bartels MC, van Rij G: Implantation of Artisan toric phakic intraocular lenses for the correction of astigmatism and spherical errors in patients with keratoconus. J Refract Surg 2005;21: 218–222.

42 Güell JL, Morral M, Gris O, et al: Five-year follow up of 399 phakic Artisan-Verisyse implantation for myopia, hyperopia and/or astigmatism. Ophthalmology 2008;115:1002–1012.

43 Budo C, Hessloehl JC, Izak M, et al: Multicenter study of the Artisan phakic intraocular lens. J Cataract Refract Surg 2000;26:1163–1171.

44 Stulting RD, John ME, Maloney RK, US Verisyse Study Group: Three year result of Artisan/Verisyse phakic intraocular lens implantation results of the United States Food and Drug Administration Clinical Trial. Ophthalmology 2008;115:464–472.

45 Pop M, Payette Y: Initial results of endothelial cell counts after Artisan lens for phakic eyes: an evaluation of the United States Food and drug Administration OPHTEC Study. Ophthalmology 2004; 111:309–317.

46 Maloney RK, Nguyen LH, John ME: Artisan phakic intraocular lens for myopia: short-term results of a prospective, multicenter study. Ophthalmology 2002; 109:1631–1641.

47 Gimbel HV, Ziemba SL: Management of myopic astigmatism with phakic intraocular lens implantation. J Cataract Refract Surg 2002;28:883–886.

48 Uusitalo RJ, Aine E, Sen NH, et al: Implantable contact lens for high myopia. J Cataract Refract Surg 2002;28:29–36.

49 Pesando PM, Ghiringhello MP, Di Meglio G, Fanton G: Posterior chamber intraocular lens (ICL) for hyperopia: ten-year follow-up. J Cataract Refract Surg 2007;33:1579–1584.

50 Sanders DR, Doney K, Poco M: United States Food and Drug Administration clinical trial of the implantable Collamer Lens (ICL) for moderate to high myopia: three-year follow-up. Ophthalmology 2004;111:1683–1692.

51 Zaldivar R, Davidorf JM, Oscherow S: Posterior chamber phakic intraocular lens for myopia of –8 to –19 diopters. J Refract Surg 1998;14:294–305.

52 Davidorf JM, Zaldivar R, Oscherow S: Posterior chamber phakic intraocular lens for hyperopia of +4 to +11 diopters. J Refract Surg 1998;14:306–311.

53 Wollensak G: Crosslinking treatment of progressive keratoconus new hope. Curr Opin Ophthalmol 2006;17:356–360.

54 Wollensak G, Spoerl E, Seiler T: Riboflavin/ultraviolet-a-induced collagen cross-linking for the treatment of keratoconus. Am J Ophthalmol 2003;135:620–627.

55 Caporossi A, Baiocchi S, Mazzotta C, et al: Para-surgical therapy for keratoconus by riboflavin-ultraviolet type A rays induced cross-linking of corneal collagen: preliminary refractive results in an Italian study. J Cataract Refract Surg 2006;32:837–845.

56 Tan DT, Por YM: Current treatment options for corneal ectasia. Curr Opin Ophthalmol 2007;18:284–289.

57 Kaneopollus AJ, Binder PS: Collagen cross-linking (CCL) with sequential topography-guided PRK: a temporizing alternative for keratoconus to penetrating keratoplasty. Cornea 2007;26:891–895.

58 Coskunseven E, Jankov MR II, Hafezi F: Contralateral eye study of collagen cross-linking with riboflavin and UVA irradiation in patients with keratoconus. J Refract Surg 2009;25:371–376.

59 Chan CCK, Sharma M, Boxer Wachler BS: Effect of interior-segment Intacts with and without C3-R on keratoconus. J Cataract Refract Surg 2007;33:75–80.

60 Kamburoglu G, Ertan A: Intacts implantation with sequential collagen cross-linking treatment in postoperative LASIK ectasia. J Refract Surg 2008: S726–S729.

61 Krueger RR, Kanellopoulus AJ: Stability of simultaneous topography-guided photorefractive keratectomy and riboflavin/UVA cross-linking for progressive keratoconus: case reports. J Refract Surg 2010;26:S827–S832.

62 Kymionis AE, Magarakis M, Yoo S, Pallikaris IG: Simultaneous topography-guided PRK followed by corneal collagen cross-linking for keratoconus. J Refract Surg 2009;25:S807–S811.

63 Kanellopoulos AJ: Comparison of sequential vs same day simultaneous collagen cross-linking and topography-guided PRK for treatment of keratoconus. J Refract Surg 2009;25:S812–S818.

64 Stojanovic A, Zhang J, Chen X, Nitter TA, Chen S, Wang Q: Topography-guided transepithelial surface ablation followed by corneal collagen cross-linking performed in a single combined procedure for the treatment of keratoconus and pellucid marginal degeneration. J Refract Surg 2010;26:145–152.

65 Izquierdo L Jr, Henriquez MA, McCarthy M: Artiflex phakic intraocular lens implantation after corneal collagen cross-linking in keratoconic eyes. J Refract Surg 2011;27:482–487.

66 Güell JL, Morral M, Malecaze F, et al: Collagen crosslinking and toric iris-claw phakic intraocular lens for myopic astigmatism in progressive mild to moderate keratoconus. J Cataract Refract Surg 2012;38:475–484.

67 Güell JL, Morral M, Salinas C, et al: Four-year follow up of intrastromal corneal ring segments in patients with keratoconus. J Emmetropia 2010;1:9–15.

68 Bower Wachler BS, Christie JP, Chandra NS, et al: Intacs for keratoconus. Ophthalmology 2003;110:1031–1040.

69 Guell JL, Morral M, Salinas C, et al: Intrastromal corneal ring segments to correct low myopia in eyes with irregular or abnormal topography including forme fruste keratoconus: 4-year follow-up. J Cataract Refract Surg 2010;36:1149–1155.

70 Kymionis GD, Kontadakis GA, Kounis GA, et al: Simultaneous topography-guided PRK followed by corneal collagen cross-linking for keratoconus. J Refract Surg 2009;25:S807–S811.

71 Kohnen T, Kook D, Morral M, Güell JL: Phakic intraocular lenses: part 2: results and complications. J Cataract Refract Surg 2010;36:2168–2194.

72 Güell JL, Morral M, Kook D, Kohnen T: Phakic intraocular lenses part 1: historical overview, current models, selection criteria, and surgical techniques. J Cataract Refract Surg 2010;36:1976–1993.

73 Huang D, Schallhorn SC, Sugar A, et al: Phakic intraocular lens implantation for the correction of myopia: a report by the American Academy of Ophthalmology. Ophthalmology 2009;116:2244–2258.

74 Dick HB, Budo C, Malecaze F, et al: Foldable Artiflex phakic intraocular lens for the correction of myopia: two-year follow-up results of a prospective European multicenter study. Ophthalmology 2009;116:671–677.

75 Tahzib NG, Nuijts RM, Wu WY, Budo CJ: Long-term study of Artisan phakic intraocular lens implantation for the correction of moderate to high myopia: ten-year follow-up results. Ophthalmology 2007;114:1133–1142.

76 Sanders DR, Schneider D, Martin R, et al: Toric Implantable Collamer Lens for moderate to high myopic astigmatism. Ophthalmology 2007;114:54–61.

77 Bartels MC, Santana NT, Budo C, et al: Toric phakic intraocular lens for the correction of hyperopia and astigmatism. J Cataract Refract Surg 2006;32:243–249.

78 Alfonso JF, Fernández-Vega L, Lisa C, et al: Collagen copolymer toric posterior chamber phakic intraocular lens in eyes with keratoconus. J Cataract Refract Surg 2010;36:906–916.

79 Alfonso JF, Palacios A, Montés-Micó R: Myopic phakic STAAR collamer posterior chamber intraocular lenses for keratoconus. J Refract Surg 2008;24:867–874.

80 Kamiya K, Shimizu K, Ando W, et al: Phakic toric Implantable Collamer Lens for the correction of high myopic astigmatism in eyes with keratoconus. J Refract Surg 2008;24:840–842.

81 Venter J: Artisan phakic intraocular lens in patients with keratoconus. J Refract Surg 2009;25:759–764.

82 Moshirfar M, Grégoire FJ, Mirzaian G, et al: Use of Verisyse iris-supported phakic intraocular lens for myopia in keratoconic patients. J Cataract Refract Surg 2006;32:1227–1232.

83 Budo C, Bartels MC, van Rij G: Implantation of Artisan toric phakic intraocular lenses for the correction of astigmatism and spherical errors in patients with keratoconus. J Refract Surg 2005;21:218–222.

84 Kymionis GD, Grentzelos MA, Karavitaki AE, et al: Combined corneal collagen cross-linking and posterior chamber toric implantable collamer lens implantation for keratoconus. Ophthalmic Surg Lasers Imaging 2011;17:42.

85 Van der Heijde GL: Some optical aspects of implantation of an intraocular lens in a myopia eye. Eur J Implant Refract Surg 1989;1:245–248.

86 Budo C, Hessloehl JC, Izak M, et al: Multicenter study of the Artisan phakic intraocular lens. J Cataract Refract Surg 2000;26:1163–1171.

87 Saxena R, Boekhoorn SS, Mulder PG, et al: Long-term follow-up of endothelial cell change after Artisan phakic intraocular lens implantation. Ophthalmology 2008;115:608–613.

88 Benedetti S, Casamenti V, Benedetti M: Long-term endothelial changes in phakic eyes after Artisan intraocular lens implantation to correct myopia: five-year study. J Cataract Refract Surg 2007; 33:784–790.

Jose L. Güell
Instituto Microcirugía Ocular, Universidad Autónoma de Barcelona
Josep Maria Lladó, 3
ES–08035 Barcelona (Spain)
E-Mail guell@imo.es

Güell JL (ed): Cataract. ESASO Course Series. Basel, Karger, 2013, vol 3, pp 116–128
DOI: 10.1159/000350913

Laser Corneal Refractive Surgery: An Update

Daniel Elies · Jose L. Güell · Paula Verdaguer · Oscar Gris · Felicidad Manero

Instituto Microcirugía Ocular, Universidad Autónoma de Barcelona, Barcelona, Spain

Abstract

Lamellar corneal surgery for the correction of refractive errors has been evolving for more than 60 years. LASIK (laser-assisted in situ keratomileusis) is a well-known procedure for correction of different refractive defects as myopia, hyperopia and astigmatism. It is the most widely used refractive surgical technique due to its safety and effectiveness, quick visual recovery, and minimal side effects. The introduction of wavefront-guided laser technology into the field of refractive surgery in 1999 represented a significant advancement in ophthalmology, allowing an optimized correction not only of spherocylindrical errors but also of higher-order aberrations. Femtosecond lasers were introduced in the place of mechanical microkeratomes, and in the past few years have rapidly become accepted as a safe and effective way to create flaps for LASIK, various corneal transplant configurations, and intracorneal channels for treating ectatic corneal disorders. The ultimate goal has been to create an intrastromal lenticule that can be removed in one piece manually, thereby avoiding the need for photoablation by an excimer laser. The results of the first prospective trials of this technique have been reported.

Copyright © 2013 S. Karger AG, Basel

Introduction

Lamellar corneal surgery for the correction of refractive errors has been evolving for more than 60 years, since Dr. Barraquer began developing lamellar corneal surgery in 1948 [1–4]. Fundamentally, refractive lamellar corneal surgery attempts to remove, add, or modify the corneal stroma so that the radius of curvature of the anterior corneal interface is changed as desired.

LASIK (laser-assisted in situ keratomileusis) is a well-known procedure for correction of different refractive defects as myopia, hyperopia and astigmatism [5, 6]. Current LASIK uses a hinged flap avoiding corneal instability; it precisely sculpts the stromal bed, sidestepping the pain, corneal haze and regression.

Principles, Techniques and Results

LASIK is typically performed in two stages and with two laser platforms: flap creation with a microkeratome or femtosecond laser followed by stromal refractive ablation with the excimer laser.

Excimer laser-based refractive surgery procedures have been performed in millions of people worldwide to improve vision and quality of life. In combination with more sensitive preoperative screening and wavefront-driven treatment profiles, the current generation of excimer laser platforms is safer, more precise and more predictable than ever before [7, 8].

The introduction of wavefront-guided (WFG) laser technology into the field of refractive surgery in 1999 represented a significant advancement in ophthalmology, allowing an optimized correction not only of spherocylindrical errors but also of higher-order aberrations [8–10]. WFG LASIK is based on aberrometry measurements. The treatment is customized to each individual eye's mix of lower- and higher-order aberrations. WFG treats the patient's phoropter-derived sphere and cylinder and places additional pulses in the peripheral cornea based on the preoperative corneal keratometry values in an attempt to maintain the cornea's natural aspheric shape and minimize the induction of spherical aberration [11–13]. Both methods produce very good outcomes.

Femtosecond lasers were introduced in the place of mechanical microkeratomes and in the past few years have rapidly become accepted as a safe and effective way to create flaps for LASIK, various corneal transplant configurations, and intracorneal channels for treating ectatic corneal disorders.

The principal application for the femtosecond laser is flap creation during LASIK [14, 15]. When the femtosecond laser is used, flap thickness is not affected by preoperative corneal curvature, corneal thickness, translation speed, or intraocular pressure. The flaps are clear, without debris, minimizing the risk of infection and diffuse lamellar keratitis. The flap shape is planar, inducing minimal aberrations and the flap architecture practically eliminates epithelial ingrowth and diminishes the occurrence of severe dry eye [16, 17].

Nowadays, we can use the femtosecond laser procedure to perform the key steps in the cataract surgery procedure. Cataract surgeons are adopting femtosecond technology to perform laser capsulotomy, lens fragmentation, clear cornea incisions and limbal relaxing incisions.

The combination of precise refractive femtosecond laser technology and lenticule extraction marks the start of a new era in refractive surgery.

Since femtosecond lasers were first introduced into refractive surgery, the ultimate goal has been to create an intrastromal lenticule that can be removed in one piece manually, thereby avoiding the need for photoablation by an excimer laser.

The VisuMax system is designed for coupling of the femtosecond laser source to the cornea with minimal tissue distortion and rapid high-precision femtosecond pulse placement.

Refractive lenticule extraction (ReLEx) is a new application that allows surgeons to perform complete laser vision correction procedures using only one laser platform. This procedure simplifies corneal refractive laser surgery because the corrective lenticule and the overlying corneal flap are created in one step using one laser. The refraction is corrected by creating an intrastromal lenticule with the femtosecond laser in the intact cornea and in a shape corresponding to the desired refractive correction.

Following the successful implementation of FLEx (femtosecond lenticule extraction), a new procedure called small incision lenticule extraction (SMILE) was developed. This procedure involves passing a dissector through a small (2–3 mm) incision to separate the lenticular interfaces and allow the lenticule to be removed, thus eliminating the need to create a flap. The results of the first prospective trials of SMILE have been reported, and there are now more than 50 surgeons routinely performing this procedure worldwide.

There are two main methods to create a corneal flap; a microkeratome with a metal blade, or a femtosecond laser such as the VisuMax (Carl Zeiss Meditec, Jena, Germany, 2007) [18].

VisuMax is a high repetition rate femtosecond system (500 kHz repetition rate), with a wavelength of 1,043 nm and 580 fs pulse duration. This technology allows for the patient to maintain visual sight during the entire procedure. This provides maximum comfort and allows you to see throughout the entire procedure, unlike with microkeratomes or other femtosecond lasers, where the patient's vision is 'blacked out' for a while and patients have reported feeling uncomfortable pressure. Because patients retain their ability to see during the surgical procedure, they are able to actively cooperate throughout the entire laser treatment. The procedure can be continued for the second eye without moving the patient back to the observation position providing an improved workflow. The VisuMax also improves the patient experience compared with using a mechanical microkeratome or many of the femtosecond lasers employing scleral suction and flat applanation. Most femtosecond systems require high suction that causes the eye to blackout during the time taken to create the flap, greatly decreasing patient comfort and increasing the chances of sub-conjunctival hemorrhages. In contrast, the intraocular pressure increase with the VisuMax is low enough for the patient to see throughout the procedure. The combination of using a curved contact glass rather than a flat contact system and corneal suction instead of scleral suction means that the intraocular pressure rise during the procedure is generally below 90 or 100 mm Hg. One study compared the intraocular pressure rise during flap creation with the VisuMax, IntraLase and Da Vinci femtosecond laser systems. The mean intraocular pressure during flap creation was reported to be 84.9 ± 7.3 mm Hg for the VisuMax, 180.6 ± 21.6 mm Hg

for the IntraLase, and 150.9 ± 17.2 mm Hg for the Da Vinci [19].

The Carl Zeiss Meditec MEL 80 Excimer Laser System is designed to make the correction of vision defects, with extremely fast ablation, customized treatment planning with the optional CRS Master, the high-performance eye tracker system and the 'eye registration' torsion compensation system. The exceptionally fast MEL 80's short ablation time (250 Hz repetition rate) reduces procedure time for greater patient comfort, and shortened stromal exposure time means faster visual recovery and better ablation. Its very small (0.7-mm) spot permits the finest corrections without losing the benefits of smooth ablation and the two specially optimized ablation profiles (TS and ASA) to choose from help produce excellent results. The MEL 80 excimer laser has an active eye tracker with excellent feedback times and an ultrarapid iris recognition camera catching both pupil and limbus provides exact positioning during the laser treatment.

The main characteristics of the VisuMax system are as follows:

- The VisuMax coupling contact glass interface with the cornea is curved, thus leading to very little corneal distortion when securing full corneal surface contact.
- Corneal coupling of the contact glass is achieved with very low suction force applied through specifically designed suction ports that are applied to the peripheral cornea/limbus, but not the corneal conjunctiva/sclera. This low suction coupling force minimizes corneal distortion.
- Each contact glass is individually calibrated by a built-in optical coherence imagine system, thus compensating for individual differences in contact glass geometry that are inevitable in serial production.
- The optical beam path system coupled to the contact glass is suspended on a fulcrum. The fulcrum, together with a continuous force-feedback servo control for patient bed height, produces a system delivering a constant force

of the contact glass onto the cornea. This constant force minimizes changes in corneal distortion that may occur with patient head movement during the femtosecond cutting process.

- The optical system delivering the femtosecond beam is designed with very high numerical aperture optics, thus allowing for very tight concentration of femtosecond energy, very little collateral energy dissipation and high femtosecond spot placement accuracy.
- The laser-tissue interaction dynamics are optimized for speed with a repetition rate of 500 kHz, which minimizes treatment time and achieves the critical refractive cuts in a short enough time to reduce the chances of eye or patient movements during this phase of the cutting.

The most recent advance by Carl Zeiss Meditec Inc. goes beyond the flap's creation with a curved ocular interface to techniques that use the femtosecond laser for an all-in-one refractive procedure called ReLEx (for ReLEx) with the VisuMax femtosecond laser. In that new procedure, no 193-nm excimer laser is needed. The ReLEx technique can conceptually correct any refractive error – nowadays, simple myopia and compound myopic astigmatism.

ReLEx encompasses two different approaches, the first is the FLEx procedure [20, 21], the second approach to ReLEx is the small-incision lenticule extraction or SMILE technique [22, 23]. During the FLEx approach, the femtosecond laser makes essentially two passes. The first or posterior pass of the femtosecond laser creates the posterior surface of the lenticule that will be extracted, while the second or anterior pass of the laser accomplishes three goals: the flap's side cuts, the side cut to lenticule edge pass effectively creating the peripheral stromal bed, and the anterior surface of the lenticule that will be extracted. The FLEx procedure diverges from traditional LASIK in that, instead of the excimer laser being used for the 'refractive step', the femtosecond laser creates a lenticule of corneal tissue for removal to cause the refractive change. In this setting, the procedure is reminiscent of automated lamellar keratoplasty. The major difference is that the refractive predictability and corneal shape modification capability is on par with excimer-based corneal refractive procedures.

In the SMILE technique, rather than creating and lifting a hinged flap, the surgeon performs two passes of the femtosecond laser; as in the FLEx procedure, the first pass of the laser creates the posterior aspect of the lenticule and a peripheral stromal bed. The second pass of the femtosecond laser creates the anterior surface of the lenticule and one or two small access incisions [22, 23]. The surgeon can then dissect the remaining corneal attachments of the anterior and posterior surfaces and remove the lenticule through a small incision. Only part of the anterior flap side cut is completed to the surface, followed by removal of the lenticule through a 4- to 5-mm superior corneal tunnel.

The potential advantages of the SMILE concept are that it is less invasive, it results in less postoperative irritation due to the small epithelial cut; the loss of corneal sensibility is potentially smaller, and there is less effect on tear production because the small incision cuts fewer corneal nerves. Additionally, there is the potential for greater flap and biomechanical stability and a lower risk of corneal ectasia due to the preservation of continuous anterior stromal lamellae across the cornea. There are some concerns about long-term data, which are lacking. It is also currently unclear if very small refractive errors (≤ 1.00 dpt) can be precisely corrected with the ReLEx procedure, and furthermore what surgeons can achieve for the typical enhancement cases with a spherical equivalent of <1.00 dpt.

Surgical Technique

The surgery starts by managing the patient with a mild anxiolytic and sedative orally (diazepam, Valium 5 mg, Roche) 30 min before surgery. Under topical anesthesia (oxybuprocaine hydrochloride 0.4%, Prescaina, Llorens Lab) and after a povidone-iodine (Betadine) scrub of the skin and eyelids, the patients are draped with a sterile head towel, and the eyelashes are taped with a sterile tape, the patient lies down on the ergonomic pivoting patient table.

The VisuMax femtosecond ReLEx procedure starts with the application of an eyelid speculum to keep the eye open, the patient's eye is positioned under a curved contact glass interface. The contact glass is similar to a gonioscopic lens, in that it possesses a curved surface designed to couple with the cornea with only a minimal applanation force. Before coupling, the VisuMax system self-calibrates the contact glass. The eye's keratometry data are entered into the VisuMax to account for the difference between the relaxed cornea and the contact glass curvature. The contact glass is available in three sizes: small, medium, and large. The size of the contact glass is chosen depending on the white-to-white diameter. The maximum flap diameter ranges from 8.0 mm for the small contact glass to 9.5 mm for the large contact glass. For ReLEx procedure, the small contact glass is recommended.

A fully device-integrated suction system ensures that suction is only applied to the cornea during the actual laser treatment. Automatic corneal suction is continuously monitored throughout the surgery and takes only seconds longer than the actual laser incision itself. Centration is supported with several features including an internal fixation target for the patient designed to attract their attention, self-adjustment of the eye during docking to contact glass, easy to find visual axis for treatment positioning, and automated adaptation to patient eye refraction. Flap parameters that can be adjusted include the flap thickness, flap diameter, hinge width, side cut angle and hinge location.

The patient bed is moved using a joystick, which controls x, y and z, so that the eye is brought up into contact with the contact glass, while the patient is fixating on a flashing green light. Once contact is made between the cornea and the contact glass, the patient is able to see the flashing fixation target in clear focus. This aligns the eye in the primary position, allowing the bed to be raised vertically while the surgeon observes the alignment of the contact glass application through the operating microscope, and the cornea flattens in a self-centering way on the corneal vertex. When full-contact glass application is achieved, suction is applied, the eye is immobilized, and the laser is activated by the surgeon pressing on a foot pedal. A very accurately focused laser beam is guided through to the cornea, the laser beam moves across and through the cornea in a spiral manner, creating a layer of very tiny bubbles under its path. These bubbles quickly disappear, and the tissue above the bubbles becomes the corneal flap or the corneal lenticule that can be easily lifted by the surgeon.

As previously stated, the intraocular pressure increase with the VisuMax is low enough for the patient to see throughout the procedure. The low intraocular pressure increase helps during the procedure as patient anxiety remains lower as they can still see the fixation light, which in turn allows the extraocular muscles to be part of the biomechanical system to keep the eye fixated during treatment.

The design of the VisuMax also lends itself well to flap centration on the corneal vertex, which closely approximates the visual axis. The VisuMax was designed to promote centration of the system onto the corneal vertex; as the patient fixates on a flashing light and the system uses a curved contact glass, the vertex of the cornea fits naturally into the vertex of the contact glass guided by the patient's sight. The VisuMax, as other femtosecond lasers, provides flexible incision geometry, so the vertical cut (90–110°) fits perfectly on the cornea minimizing the risk of postoperative displacement, striae or folds, thickness of the flap from 80 µm, and the diameter and hinge position of the flap. Intuitive software makes it possible to conveniently adjust all patient-specific treatment parameters. The VisuMax produces a very thin layer of opaque bubble layer, which we

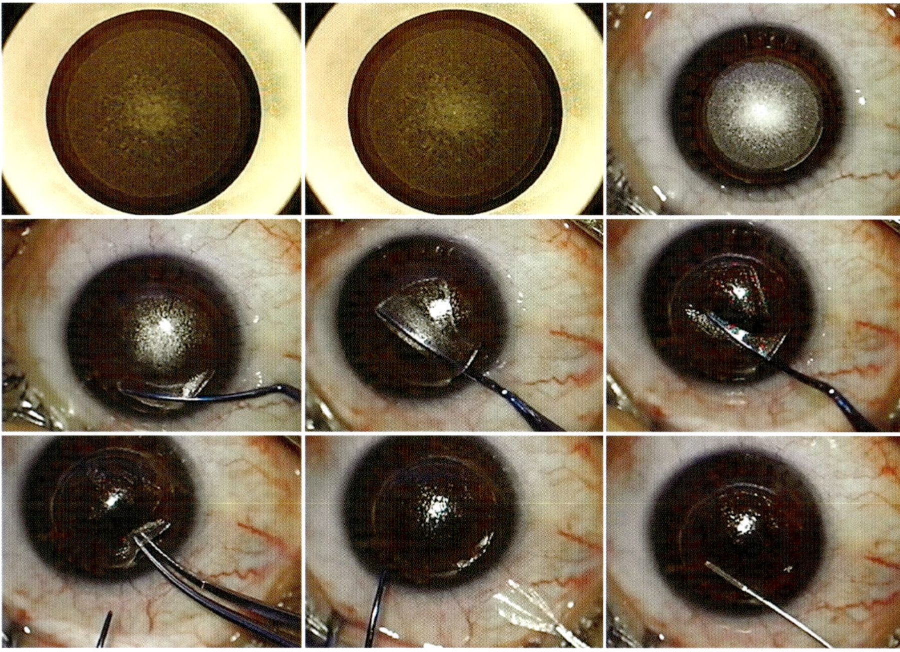

Fig. 1. Steps of the procedure of SMILE.

have found dissipates in the time between ReLEx creation and the end of the whole procedure when the patient gets up.

In the FLEx and SMILE procedures, the VisuMax is first used to remove a precise refractive lenticule from the cornea by laying down pulses that separate the posterior part of the lenticule from the stroma. In the second step, the VisuMax is used to lay down pulses that separate the anterior surface, or upper cut, of the lenticule from the stroma. The upper cut of the lenticule is extended a fraction of a millimeter beyond the edge required for the lenticule, thus serving as the flap. In a further step, the flap side cut is then created to make a hinged flap. The flap is lifted and the lenticule is extracted from the stroma. The flap is then replaced. The tissue that otherwise would have been ablated by the excimer laser is removed physically and intact in the FLEx procedure, which entails lenticule extraction rather than tissue ablation. FLEx represents the first all-in-one procedure that uses only the femtosecond laser to complete all steps in LASIK. SMILE takes this whole process a step further. Instead of making a complete flap side cut, only a small incision is created, and the flap is never lifted. Instead, the lenticule is extracted from within the cornea from a small incision (fig. 1). This virtually eliminates flap displacement in SMILE procedures, and there is little risk of the flap dislocating with trauma to the eye at a later point. Additional benefits may include reduction of dry eye problems and improvements in corneal biomechanical stability.

The entire procedure took relatively constant 50–55 s, independent of the refractive error to be corrected, which is an advantage at the time of evaluating the results postoperatively. The shape of the lenticule generated was designed to correct for refractive errors. In all cases, the anterior surface of the lenticule was 100 μm deep, and the

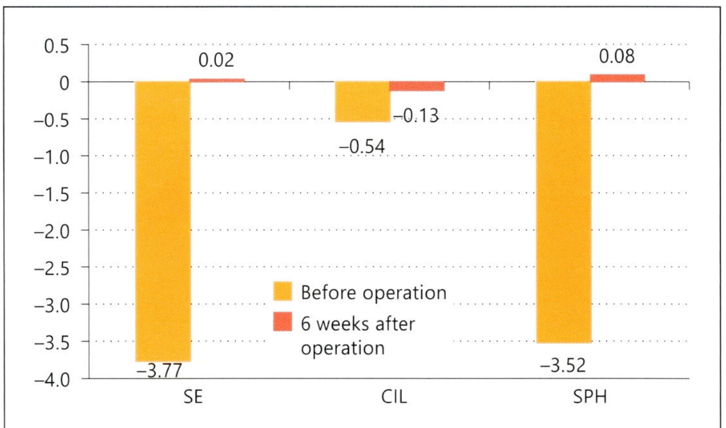

Fig. 2. Evolution of pre and post FLEx spherical equivalent, cylinder and sphere.

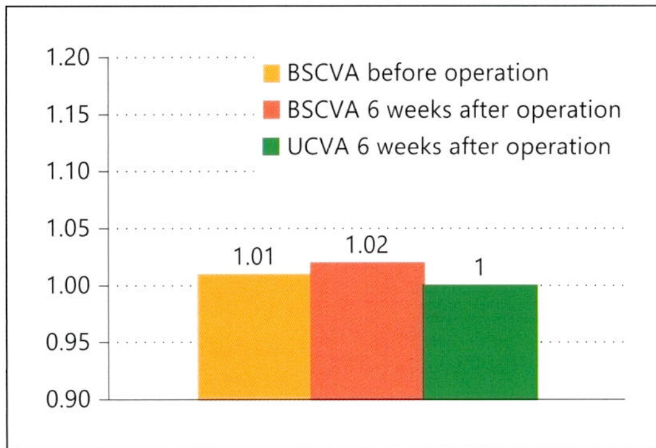

Fig. 3. Evolution of pre and post FLEx BSCVA and UCVA.

maximum diameter of the first cleavage plane, 6.0 mm. For technical reasons, astigmatism corrections result in an oval posterior surface of the lenticule. Thus, the cleavage plane diameter was 6.0 mm in the flat axis and smaller (depending on the amount of astigmatism corrected) in the steep axis. Although the lenticule side cut is always circular and intersects the plane of the lenticule, the steeper curvature defines the optical zone size (lenticule side cut diameter). For all myopic corrections, the optical zone size was 6.0 mm. The spot-and-track spacing for the cleavage plane

which defines the posterior surface of the lenticule was slightly higher than the spot-and-track spacing for the cleavage plane which defines the anterior surface of the lenticule (i.e. the cap). The posterior part of the lenticule was created by laser scanning in spirals from the center of the pupil to the periphery of the optical zone. The anterior part of the lenticule was created by laser scanning in spirals from the periphery to the center of the pupil. All passes and spot-and-track distance changes were automatically performed by the laser software and hardware with no user intervention.

Our standard postoperative treatment is antibiotic and steroid drops (Tobradex, Alcon) t.i.d. during a week and preservative-free artificial tears five times a day for almost a month.

In our center, we have performed surgery using the FLEx technique in 36 eyes of 18 patients (15 females and 3 males). The mean age was 32.0 years (21–42), the mean preoperative spherical equivalent was –3.77 dpt (–1.75 to –6.75), whereas the mean cylinder resulted in –0.54 (0 to –1.5), and the mean sphere was –3.52 dpt (–1.75 to –4.75). The mean preoperative best spectacle-corrected visual acuity (BSCVA) was 1.01 (0.8–1.2). We have reported some complications after the surgery: 1 patient (2 eyes) had subclinical stromal edema during the first 3 days, and

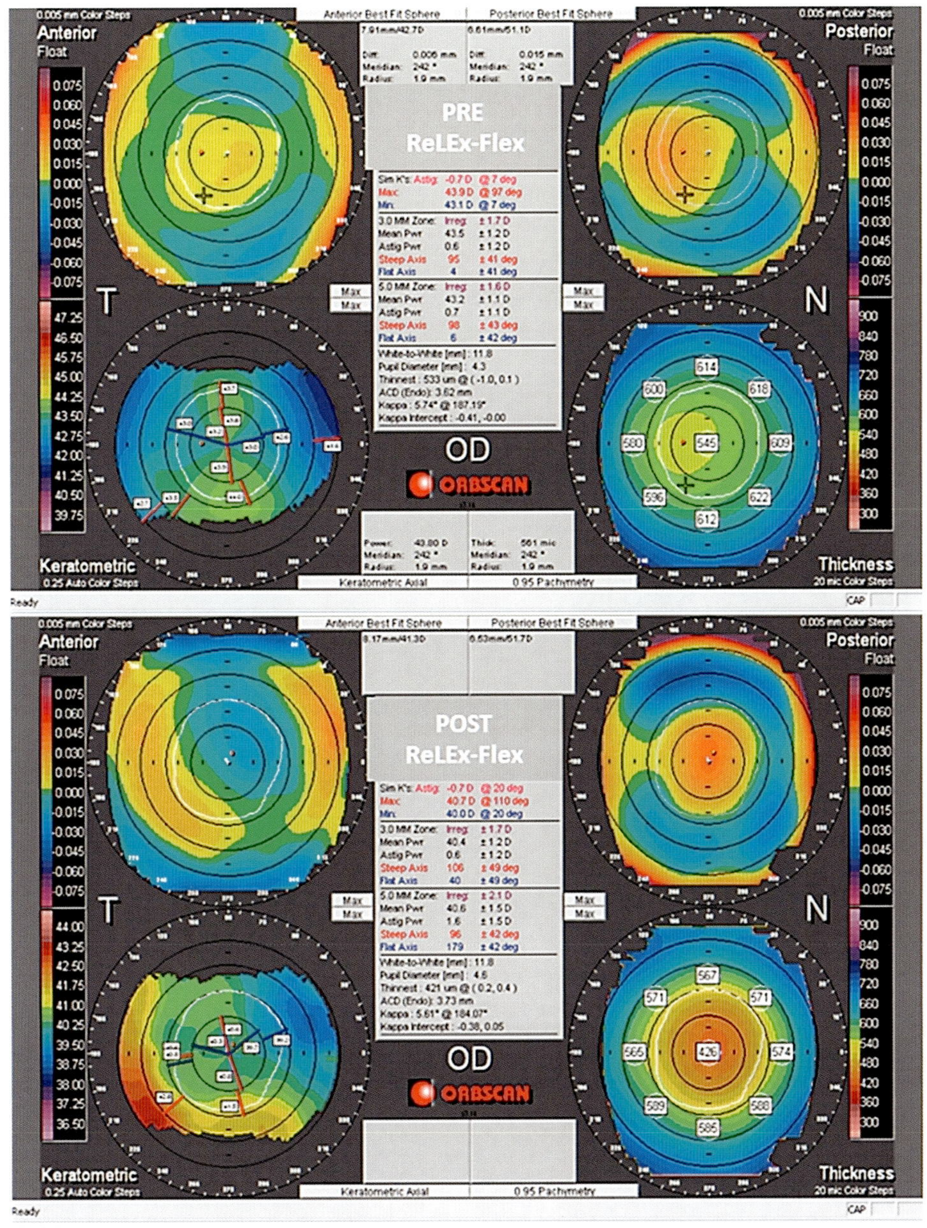

Fig. 4. Orbscan (Orbtek Inc.) corneal topography pre and post ReLEx-FLEx.

1 eye had superior decentration without subjective symptoms. Six weeks after the surgery, the spherical equivalent was 0.02, the cylinder –0.13, the sphere decrease 0.08, the uncorrected visual acuity 1.00 and the BSCVA 1.02 (fig. 2–5).

We also have experience with the SMILE technique. The initial group was the following: 14 eyes of 7 patients have been operated on (4 females and 3 males). The mean age was 36.4 years (29–46), the mean cylinder before the

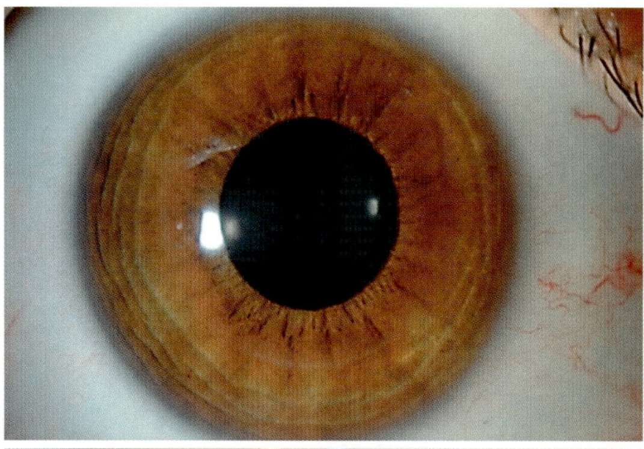

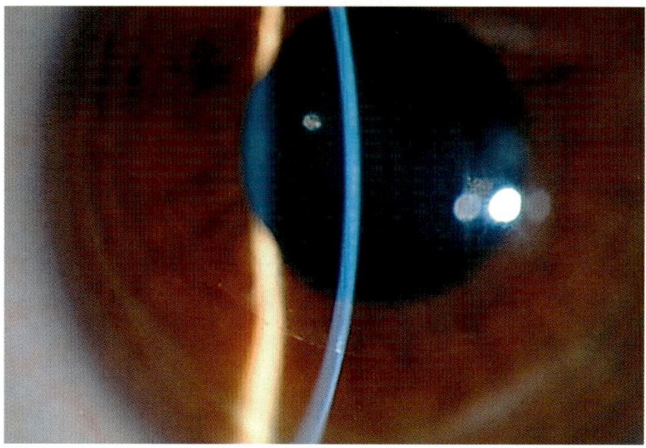

Fig. 5. Post FLEx anterior segment photo.

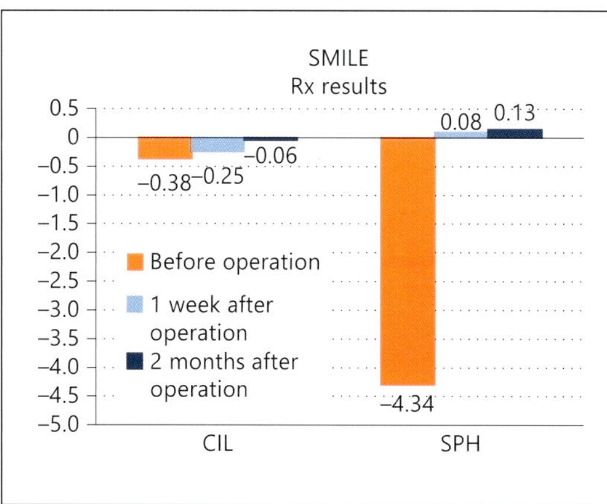

Fig. 6. Evolution of pre and post SMILE cylinder and sphere.

surgery was −0.38 dpt (0 to −0.75) and the mean sphere was −4.34 (−1.75 to −7.25). The mean BSCVA resulted in 1.05 (1–1.2), and the mean topographic K was 42.29 (41.2–43.3). All patients were operated on with the SMILE technique. One week after the surgery, the mean cylinder was −0.25, the mean sphere was 0.08 and the mean topographic K was 38.02 (fig. 6). One month after the surgery, the mean K was 40.23. Two months after the surgery, the mean cylinder reduced to −0.06, the mean sphere was 0.13, the mean BSCVA improved to 0.91, the mean uncorrected visual acuity was 0.9 and the mean topographic K resulted in 40.1 (fig. 7, 8).

The OSI index (OQAS Scattering Index) was 2.77 one week after the surgery, 2.92 one month and 2.75 2 months after the surgery (fig. 9). Both BSCVA and the OSI came back to the preoperative level or better around 6 months after the surgery.

The full group of our study is being evaluated, and the report has been submitted for publication in the *Journal of Cataract and Refractive Surgery*.

Therefore, these new femtosecond intrastromal lenticule procedures offer a number of potential advantages:

1 More accurate and repeatable tissue removal independent of prescription treated.
2 Increased biomechanical integrity of the postoperative cornea (fig. 10).
3 Reduction in postoperative dry eye symptoms and recovery.

Taking into account the higher frequency of complications, especially epithelial ingrowth, after LASIK regressions and mostly when the first cut was made by a mechanical microkeratome, another very useful approach per reLASIK is to prepare a vertical cut with the femtosecond laser inside the old cut, to 'cleanly' access the interface. This is becoming our standard approach for retreatment.

Until now, the surgeries we have performed with FLEx in patients with moderate myopia have

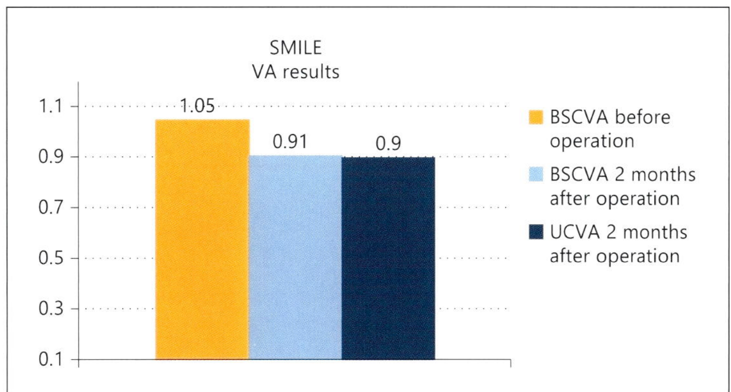

Fig. 7. Evolution of pre and post SMILE VA.

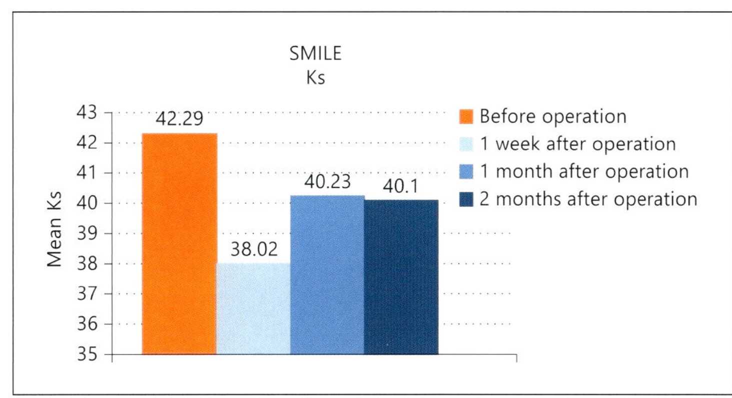

Fig. 8. Evolution of pre and post SMILE Ks.

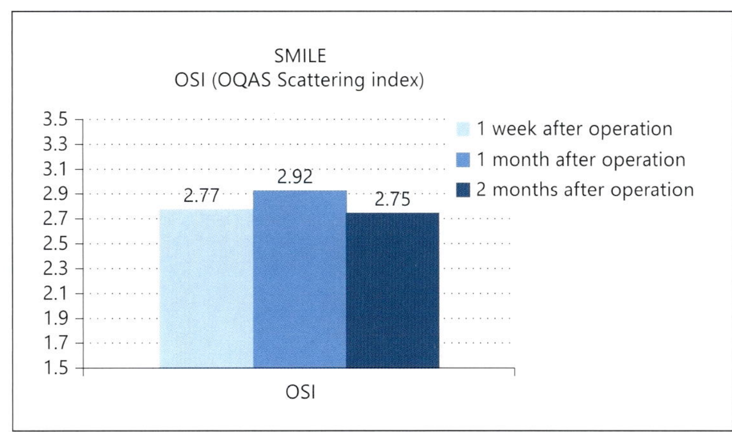

Fig. 9. Evolution of OSI index (OQAS Scattering index) after the SMILE surgery.

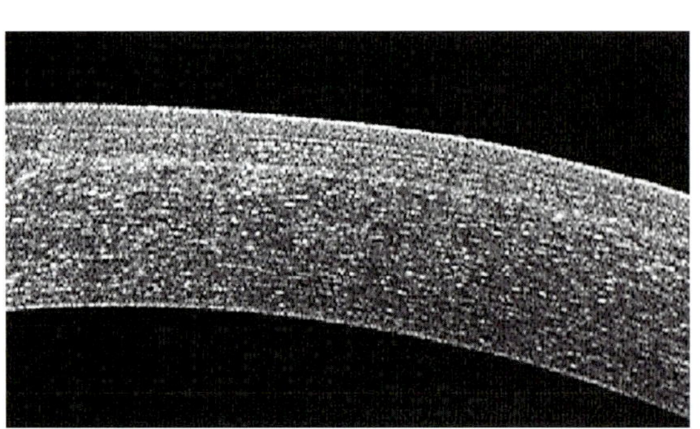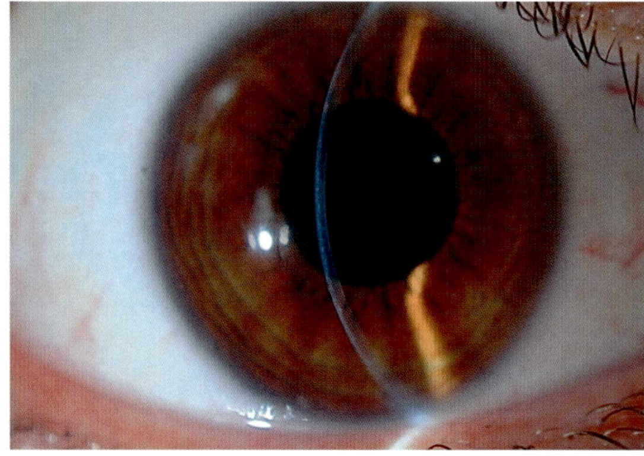

Fig. 10. Post SMILE anterior segment photo and OCT.

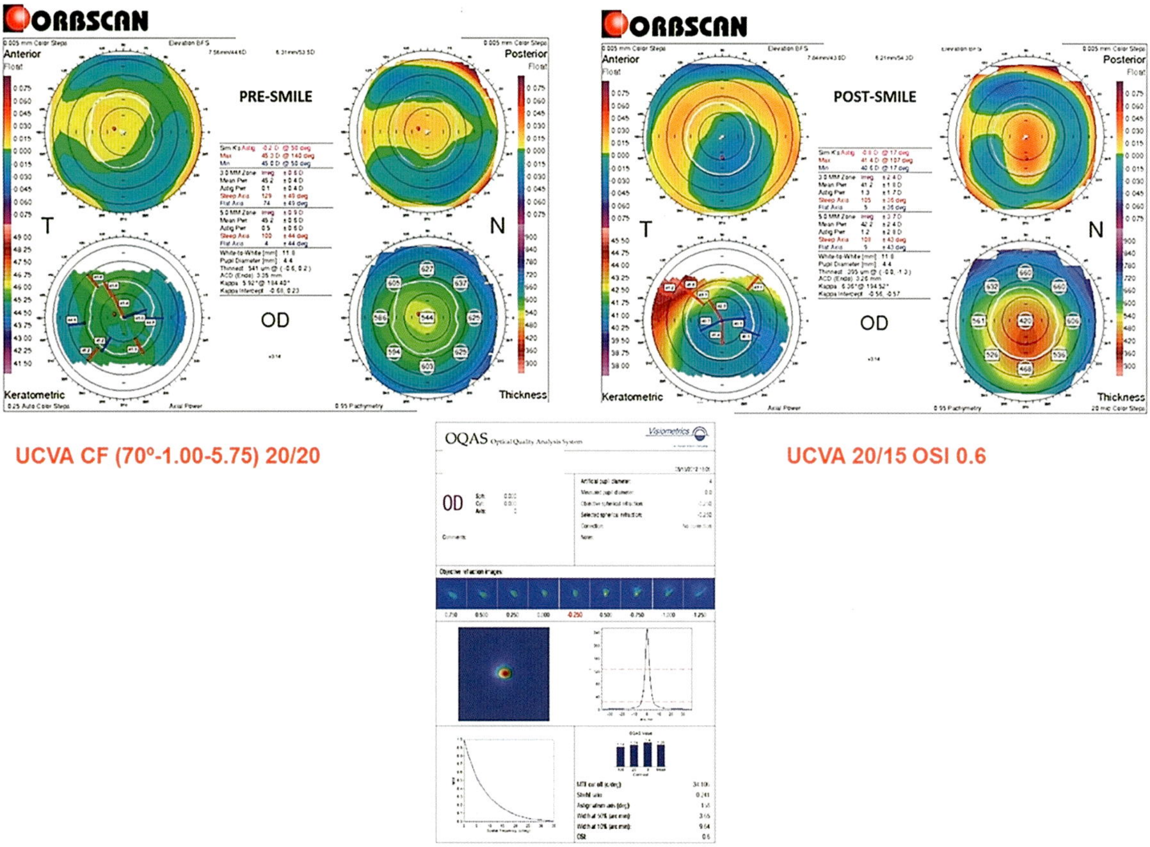

Fig. 11. Orbscan (Orbtek Inc.) corneal topography pre and post SMILE. OSI index (OQAS Scattering index) after the SMILE surgery of this patient.

Elies · Güell · Verdaguer · Gris · Manero

been associated with high precision, similar to other published data [20, 21] (fig. 11). Although no patient required it in our FLEX series, enhancement may be performed when necessary using the excimer laser after manual lifting of the flap.

The refractive results in published studies are excellent [20, 21]. In the study by Shah et al. [23], 91% of eyes were within ±0.50 dpt of the target refraction at 6 months. The refraction in those patients remained very stable postoperatively, and the authors did not describe any significant complications, apart from mild dryness, contact glass loss of suction in one eye (1.8%) and slight corneal cap edema the day before in <10% of the eyes, which spontaneously resolved.

There are likely advantages to using a femtosecond laser for refractive correction over using an excimer laser. Although modern excimer lasers compensate for the peripheral undercorrection and central overcorrection observed with an earlier generation of excimer lasers, the femtosecond laser is less affected by peripheral energy loss as it cuts the refractive lenticule, as likely occurs with an excimer laser. Furthermore, excimer laser results depend on corneal hydration characteristics and environmental conditions. It is unlikely that this would be the case with femtosecond lasers. The published results, even without nomogram correction, are comparable to those of modern excimer lasers. In contrast, excimer lasers required large nomogram correction to achieve consistent results, irrespective of the refractive error.

Conclusion

LASIK is the most widely used refractive surgical technique due to its safety and effectiveness, quick visual recovery, and minimal side effects.

The VisuMax in the 'all-in-one' bladeless femtosecond LASIK provides very high accuracy and reproducibility and excellent visual outcomes at 6-month follow-up. An all-in-one femtosecond procedure (FLEx) or SMILE techniques could lead to improvement in corneal refractive surgery as they induce less impact on the biomechanics of the cornea, and carry little risk of ocular trauma with the advantage of the simplicity of the solid-state femtosecond laser itself. Nevertheless, we must wait for further studies, longer follow-ups as well as improvements in low ametropia correction.

References

1 Barraquer JI: Queratoplastia refractiva. Estudios Inform OftalInst Barraquer 1949;10:2–21.
2 Barraquer JI: Method for cutting lamellar grafts in frozen corneas: new orientations for refractive surgery. Arch Soc Am Ophthalmol 1958;1:237.
3 Barraquer JI: Keratomileusis. Int Surg 1967;48:103–117.
4 Barraquer JI: Results of myopic keratomileusis. J Refract Surg 1987;3:98–101.
5 Pallikaris IG, Papatzanaki ME, Stathi EZ, Frenschock O, Georgiadis A: Laser in situ keratomileusis. Lasers Surg Med 1990;10:463–468.
6 Güell JL, Muller A: Laser in situ keratomileusis (LASIK) for myopia from –7 to –18 diopters. J Refract Surg 1996;12: 222–228.
7 Perez-Straziota CE, Randleman JB, Stulting RD: Visual acuity and higher-order aberrations with wavefront-guided and wavefront-optimized laser in situ keratomileusis. J Cataract Refract Surg 2010;36:437–441.
8 Moshirfar M, Schliesser JA, Chang JC, et al: Visual outcomes after wavefront-guided photorefractive keratectomy and wavefront-guided laser in situ keratomileusis: prospective comparison. J Cataract Refract Surg 2010;36:1336–1343.
9 Keir NJ, Simpson T, Jones LW, Fonn D: Wavefront-guided LASIK for myopia: effect on visual acuity, contrast sensitivity, and higher order aberrations. J Refract Surg 2009;25:524–533.
10 Schallhorn SC, Venter JA: One-month outcomes of wavefront-guided LASIK for low to moderate myopia with the VISX STAR S4 laser in 32,569 eyes. J Refract Surg 2009;25(suppl 7):S634–S641.
11 Alió JL, Montés-Mico R: Wavefront-guided versus standard LASIK enhancement for residual refractive errors. Ophthalmology 2006;113:191–197.
12 Jabbur NS, Kraff C, VisxWavefront Study Group: Wavefront-guided laser in situ keratomileusis using the WaveScan system for correction of low to moderate myopia with astigmatism: 6-month results in 277 eyes. J Cataract Refract Surg 2005;31:1493–1501.

13 Kim TI, Yang SJ, Tchah H: Bilateral comparison of wavefront-guided versus conventional laser in situ keratomileusis with Bausch and Lomb Zyoptix. J Refract Surg 2004;20:432–438.

14 Slade SG, Durrie DS, Binder PS: A prospective, contralateral eye study comparing thin-flap LASIK (sub-Bowman keratomileusis) with photorefractive keratectomy. Ophthalmology 2009;116: 1075–1082.

15 Binder PS: Femtosecond applications for anterior segment surgery. Eye Contact Lens 2010;36:282–285.

16 Durrie DS, Kezirian GM: Femtosecond laser versus mechanical keratome flaps in wavefront-guided laser in situ keratomileusis: prospective contralateral eye study. J Cataract Refract Surg 2005; 31:120–126.

17 Kezirian GM, Stonecipher KG: Comparison of the IntraLase femtosecond laser and mechanical keratomes for laser in situ keratomileusis. J Cataract Refract Surg 2004;30:804–811.

18 Reinstein DZ, Archer TJ, Gobbe M, Johnson N: Accuracy and reproducibility of artemis central flap thickness and visual outcomes of LASIK with the Carl Zeiss MeditecVisuMax femtosecond laser and MEL 80 excimer laser platforms. J Refract Surg 2010;26:107–119.

19 Grabner G: Femtosecond to fully replace microkeratome. Ophthalmol Times 2008.

20 Blum M, Kunert K, Schröder M, Sekundo W: Femtosecond lenticule extraction for the correction of myopia: preliminary 6-month results. Graefes Arch Clin Exp Ophthalmol 2010;248:1019–1027.

21 Sekundo W, Kunert K, Russmann C, Gille A, Bissmann W, Stobrawa G, Sticker M, Bischoff M, Blum M: First efficacy and safety study of femtosecond lenticule extraction for the correction of myopia: six-month results. J Cataract Refract Surg 2008;34:1513–1520, erratum in J Cataract Refract Surg 2008;34:1819.

22 Sekundo W, Kunert KS, Blum M: Small incision corneal refractive surgery using the small incision lenticule extraction (SMILE) procedure for the correction of myopia and myopic astigmatism: results of a 6 month prospective study. Br J Ophthalmol 2011;95:335–339.

23 Shah R, Shah S, Sengupta S: Results of small incision lenticule extraction: all-in-one femtosecond laser refractive surgery. J Cataract Refract Surg 2011;37: 127–137.

Daniel Elies
Instituto Microcirugía Ocular
Universidad Autónoma de Barcelona
Josep Maria Lladó 3, ES–08035 Barcelona (Spain)
E-Mail elies@imo.es

Güell JL (ed): Cataract. ESASO Course Series. Basel, Karger, 2013, vol 3, pp 129–136
DOI: 10.1159/000350914

Intracorneal Refractive Surgery: Lenses and Ring Segments

Ioannis G. Pallikaris

Department of Ophthalmology, Medical School, University of Crete, Heraklion, Greece

Abstract

Intracorneal refractive surgery includes intracorneal inlay implantation for presbyopia reversal and intracorneal ring segment (ICRS) implantation, originally designed to treat low to moderate myopia and currently used to treat ectatic corneal disorders such as post-LASIK corneal ectasia, pellucid marginal degeneration and keratoconus. The intracorneal inlay implantation procedure is a minimally invasive reversible surgical technique with encouraging clinical results. ICRS are inserted into intrastromal channels (created either manually or with femtosecond lasers) at 75% depth of the thinnest pachymetry so as to flatten the central corneal zone and improve visual acuity.

Introduction

The cornea contributes to approximately 2/3 of total refractive power of the eye, making it the most powerful refractive medium. Therefore, small changes in corneal refractive power translate into greater refractive corrections giving rise to optimum refractive outcomes. Furthermore, easy accessibility, avascularity and transparency of the cornea makes corneal refractive surgery the most popular refractive surgical approach. Cor-

neal refractive surgery can be divided into superficial corneal refractive surgery (surface ablation, LASIK, conductive keratoplasty, etc.) and intracorneal refractive surgery (intracorneal lens, corneal ring segments). This chapter will address contemporary intracorneal refractive surgery, which includes intracorneal lens (intracorneal inlay) implantation for presbyopia reversal and intracorneal ring segment (ICRS) implantation for correcting mild to moderate myopia and keratoconus rehabilitation.

Intracorneal Refractive Surgery: Intracorneal Lenses (Inlays)

The necessity to develop a minimally invasive technique for compensation of presbyopia in 45- to 60-year-old emmetropic, presbyopic patients, who are considered too old for laser corneal refractive surgery and too young for the crystalline lens extraction procedure, has led to the development of a new approach of intracorneal inlay implantation. Intracorneal lenses (inlays) are implanted under a lamellar flap or into an intrastromal corneal pocket in the nondominant eye of the patient, thus providing improved unaided near vision by various mechanisms of action. The intracorneal pocket is created either mechanically with a special microkeratome or with the femtosecond (FS) laser. Major advantages of the intracorneal lens implantation procedure are the minimally invasive nature, easy surgical technique requiring no special surgical skills, potential reversibility and the ability to combine several surgical corneal and intraocular modalities for the correction of refractive errors and presbyopia [1].

History of Intracorneal Lenses
In 1949, José Barraquer [2] first described the implantation of a synthetic lenticule inside the cornea for the correction of aphakia and high myopia. The technique was known as synthetic keratophakia, and intracorneal lenses were composed of glass and Plexiglas. High-index polymers like polymethyl methacrylate polysulfone were used as materials of intracorneal lenses due to their optical abilities in order to treat Fuch's endothelial dystrophy and high myopia [3]. Their inadequate permeability for fluids, nutrients and products of cell metabolism led to anterior stromal thinning of the cornea, stromal opacities and keratolysis.

Later on, modern intracorneal inlays were developed, and the results of the experimental use of synthetic polymers such as glyceryl methacrylate [4] and then hydrogel [5] demonstrated hydrogel to be the material of choice for intracorneal inlays. Hydrogel was semi-permeable to fluids and nutrient ingredients for the cornea, but had limited optical properties due to its low optical index of refraction. Modern inlays that have been studied in the past include Kerato-Gel (Allergan Inc., Irvine, USA) inlay made from Lidofilcon A, Chiron inlay (Bausch and Lomb, Rochester, N.Y., USA) from hydrogel material, and PermaVision Intracorneal Lens (Anamed, Lake Forest, Calif., USA) made from a hydrogel-based material called Nutrapore containing 78% water. Its mechanism of action was to alter anterior cornea's surface curvature to treat ametropia and presbyopia by creating a multifocal pattern on the tissue's surface. A similar

mechanism of action was recorded for the Intra-Lens (Lake Forest, Calif., USA) and the current Raindrop Near Vision Inlay (ReVision Optics, Lake Forest, Calif., USA). The Intracorneal Microlens (BioVision AG, Brugg, Switzerland) was a lenticule 3.0 mm in diameter and 20 μm in thickness, made from hydrogel, with an additional refractive power and central opening permitting the flow of fluids and nutrients to the anterior central cornea. This inlay was implanted into a stromal pocket created by a mechanical microkeratome. The Microlens was later named InVue, which represents the former inlay of the Flexivue™ inlay (Presbia, Amsterdam, The Netherlands).

Contemporary Intracorneal Inlays
Current intracorneal inlays for the compensation of presbyopia in emmetropic patients are utilized for investigational purposes and are not yet approved by the United States Food and Drug Administration. They consist of the KAMRA inlay (AcuFocus, Irvine, Calif., USA), the Vue+ (ReVision Optics), and the Flexivue Microlens (Presbia). Currently utilized intracorneal inlays for the treatment of presbyopia can be categorized into three groups according to their mechanisms of action: (a) Intracorneal inlays that act as small apertures increasing the depth of focus through a pinhole effect. These are made of polyvinylidine fluoride and an example is the Kamra inlay (AcuFocus). (b) Intracorneal inlays that reshape the anterior surface of the cornea, increasing its curvature, making it steeper. Those inlays are made of hydrogel, and an example is the Vue+ inlay (ReVision). (c) Intracorneal inlays that serve as a refractive addition lens, creating a bifocal optical system in the patient's cornea. They are made up of a hydrophilic acrylic material, and an example is the Flexivue Microlens (The Netherlands).

KAMRA Inlay by AcuFocus
The KAMRA inlay by AcuFocus is a small aperture corneal inlay for the treatment of presbyopia in emmetropic, presbyopic patients that utilizes

the pinhole effect to increase the depth of field by selecting central light rays only. The Kamra inlay has an outer diameter of 3.8 mm, a central annulus of 1.6 mm that serves as pinhole, and a thickness of 5 μm. It is made of biocompatible polyvinylidine fluoride material and is implanted under the LASIK flap or inside a corneal pocket at 200-μm stromal depth created by the FS laser. It has 8,400 laser-etched openings of 5.5–11.5 μm distributed in a designed pseudorandom pattern in order to allow metabolic flow to the anterior cornea. A combined implantation of the Kamra inlay with simultaneously performed LASIK to treat ametropia and presbyopia has been described. In that case, the inlay is placed under a corneal flap at a depth of 200 μm after the ablation in order to free the patient from glasses for far and near activities.

Seyeddain et al. [6] reported 2-year data on the AcuFocus inlay implanted in 32 eyes and stated that 96.9% of patients could read J3 or better in the operated eye with a mean binocular uncorrected near acuity of J1 and a mean binocular uncorrected distance visual acuity of 20/16. Yilmaz et al. [7] reported 12-month results in 39 presbyopic patients of which 12 were naturally emmetropic and 27 had emmetropia resulting from earlier hyperopic LASIK. The mean uncorrected near visual acuity (UCNA) improved from J6 preoperatively to J1+ at one-year follow-up. The mean uncorrected distance visual acuity in the operated eyes did not change significantly from the preoperative visual acuity and remained 20/20 throughout the monitoring period.

The Raindrop Near Vision Corneal Inlay, Formerly Known as the Vue+ and Presbylens (ReVision Optics)

The Raindrop Near Vision Inlay, formerly known as the Vue+ and Presbylens (ReVision Optics) has received CE Mark authorization in Europe and is currently in a phase III clinical trial in the United States. It is a permeable hydrogel lenticule with a refractive index similar to the human cornea that gently reshapes the anterior curvature of the cornea. The inlay has a diameter of 2 mm, is approximately 10 μm thick at the periphery and has a thickness from 24 to 40 μm at the central part. The inlay is inserted under either a LASIK flap or into a corneal pocket at a depth of approximately 120–130 m in the nondominant eye of the patients. Its mechanism of action includes alteration of the anterior surface of the corneal curvature, to create a multifocal cornea that improves near and intermediate visual acuity, with slightly affecting distance visual acuity. The constriction of the pupil during near tasks offers an additional pseudo-accommodative help.

Sharma et al. [8] reported results on 8 emmetropic presbyopic eyes that underwent implantation of the inlay. All eyes implanted demonstrated a 20/32 or better UCNA, 2 years postoperatively. All patients were satisfied with the outcomes of the procedure and were able to perform typical near activities without glasses. Slade [9] presented the 6-month results of Vue+ inlay implantation in natural or postrefractive emmetropic presbyopes at the ASCRS Meeting in 2010. Mean UCNA was 20/25, and no patient lost two or more lines regarding far vision. Invue lens (Biovision) is another corneal inlay which is implanted inside a corneal pocket of the nondominant eye created using a mechanical microkeratome. Bouzoukis et al. [10] reported improving near visual acuity with 20/32 UNVA in 98% of the patients.

The Flexivue Microlens (Presbia)

The Flexivue microlens is a transparent, hydrophilic disc with a 3-mm diameter and edge thickness of approximately 15 μm. The central 1.6-mm diameter of the disc is plano and the peripheral zone has an add power. The additional power available ranges from +1.5 to +3.50 dpt in 0.25 dpt increments. At the center of the disc, there is a hole 0.15 mm in diameter that permits the transfer of oxygen and nutrients of the cornea through the lens.

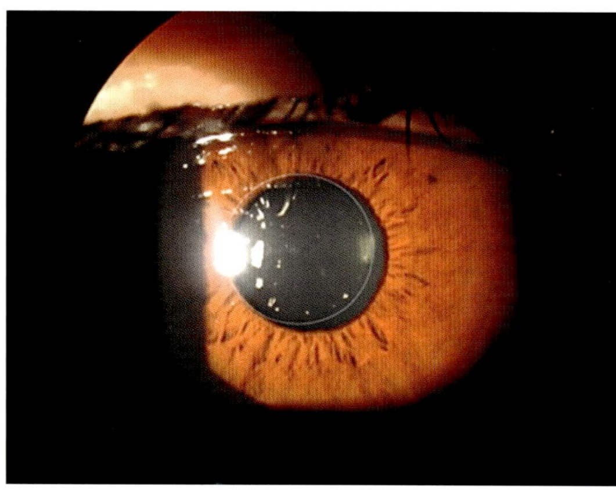

Fig. 1. The Flexivue Microlens (Presbia Inlay) inserted in the eye of a presbyopic patient.

The microlens is inserted into a stromal pocket created with the FS laser with an insertion device into the nondominant eye concentric with the estimated line of sight (fig. 1). The lens has a bifocal optical system, which acts as a modified monovision (smart monovision). During far vision, the rays pass through the central zone (plano) of the inlay without refractive effect and will be sharply focused on the retina, whereas the rays, which pass through the refractive peripheral zone, will be focused in front of the retina. During near vision, the rays which pass through the central zone will be out of focus behind the retina, and the rays which pass through the lens peripheral refractive zone will be focused on the retina. As a result, only the peripheral zone of the lens provides the near vision correction, whereas the central zone of the lens and the peripheral unaltered part of the cornea (outside the lens) do not affect the far vision.

In a recently published study of 47 emmetropic presbyopes, 12 months after surgery UCNA was 20/32 or better in 75% of operated eyes; mean uncorrected distance visual acuity (UDVA) of the operated eyes was statistically significantly decreased from 20/20 preoperatively to 20/50, whereas mean binocular UDVA did not change signi-

ficantly. Overall, higher order aberrations increased, contrast sensitivity decreased and no tissue alterations were found using corneal confocal microscopy in the operated eye [11].

Surgical Technique of Intracorneal Inlay Implantation

Intracorneal inlays may be implanted inside a corneal stromal pocket or under a lamellar corneal flap. The implantation of the intracorneal inlay inside a corneal pocket provides several advantages because the majority of peripheral corneal nerves are preserved, resulting in unaffected corneal sensitivity and potentially faster visual recovery of the patients. Pocket procedures also allow the preservation of the biomechanical properties of the cornea, offering stable mechanical stability of the tissue. Additionally, complications concerning corneal flap creation as striae, perforation of the flap and free cap are avoided. In contrast, the creation of a corneal flap permits simultaneous ablation of the stromal tissue with the excimer laser in order to treat refractive errors along with presbyopia. Also, a corneal flap allows easy manipulations during a potential reposition or removal of the inlay.

It is important to mention that since proper centration of an intracorneal inlay to treat presbyopia is vital for its better performance, the main difference from the standard procedure of creating a LASIK flap is that the irrigation of the stromal bed is avoided prior to flap repositioning in order to inhibit a potential replacement of the lenticule.

Lamellar flaps and intrastromal pockets for intracorneal inlay insertion can both be created with mechanical microkeratomes [10, 12, 13] or using an FS laser technology [14, 15]. Compared to the mechanical technique, the FS laser makes tunnel creation faster, easier and more reproducible and offers precise tunnel dimensions (width, diameter and depth) compared to manual techniques [7–15]. Thus, FS-assisted intracorneal pocket creation could increase the precision of the inlay position and result in better final visual outcomes besides improving the safety of the procedure. The development of special software for customized pockets could further simplify and increase the efficacy of the procedure. Prospective comparative studies are needed to evaluate the long-term results of the technique and optimize laser parameters. An additional advantage of the procedure is that it is not necessary to change or to add new equipment in a modern refractive surgery center, except the special injector and the mask, offering also one more application in FS laser treatments.

Complications of Intracorneal Inlay Implantation
Complications regarding the biocompatibility of the material used for the previous generation of intracorneal lenses have been described and include corneal stromal opacity, haze variants, epithelial or extracellular matrix deposits, infiltration, and keratolysis [16–18]. Confocal microscopy has been used to assess the tolerance of the intracorneal lenses in the cornea, confirming biocompatibility and showing no abnormal changes up to 1 year after the intracorneal lens implantation [19]. Modifications of the material in order to be more permeable to fluids and nutrients and byproducts of the metabolism of the tissue, along with alterations in postoperative medical treatment of the patients to include steroids and occasionally cyclosporine, have contributed to decreasing such adverse events and increasing the tolerance and stability of the outcomes. Additionally, the development of the FS lasers for the creation of the corneal tunnel has increased the predictability, speed and safety of the procedure.

Intracorneal Refractive Surgery: Ring Segments

ICRS are polymethyl methacrylate implants which are implanted intrastromally at the midperipheral cornea so as to flatten the central corneal zone. They were originally designed to treat low to moderate myopia [20] and are currently used to treat ectatic corneal disorders such as post-LASIK corneal ectasia [21], pellucid marginal degeneration [22] and keratoconus [23]. Indications for corneal ring segment insertion for the treatment of the refractive error and rehabilitation of keratectasic eyes include: low and unsatisfactory best corrected visual acuity, intolerance of contact lens wear, clear optical zone, and corneal thickness >450 μm in the area of implantation. Intrastromal ring segments are inserted into intrastromal channels (created either manually or with FS lasers) at 75% depth of the thinnest pachymetry.

Mechanism of Action
The ICRS implantation results in an arc-shortening effect and redistribution of corneal peripheral lamellae to produce flattening of the central cornea and decreasing myopia as well as astigmatism [24]. The effect is proportional to implant thickness and inversely proportional to implant diameter [25]. Ring segments have several potential advantages over other forms of refractive surgery. The ring segments can be explanted, making the refractive result of the procedure potentially reversible, and the ring segments can be replaced with ring segments of a different thickness to titrate the refractive result. The long-term results of implanting ICRS have shown effectiveness, safety and stability in correcting low myopia [26]. Unlike with surface ablation or LASIK, the central clear zone of the cornea is not directly treated. The normal cornea is generally prolate, or steeper centrally than peripherally: the central cornea profile after placement of ring segments has been shown to maintain an aspheric, prolate shape because the ring segments flatten the peripheral cornea more than the central cornea. It has been suggested that a prolate cornea may minimize visual disturbances, such as glare and halo symptoms. Because the ring segments are narrow, the overlying stroma can receive nutrients from the surrounding tissue.

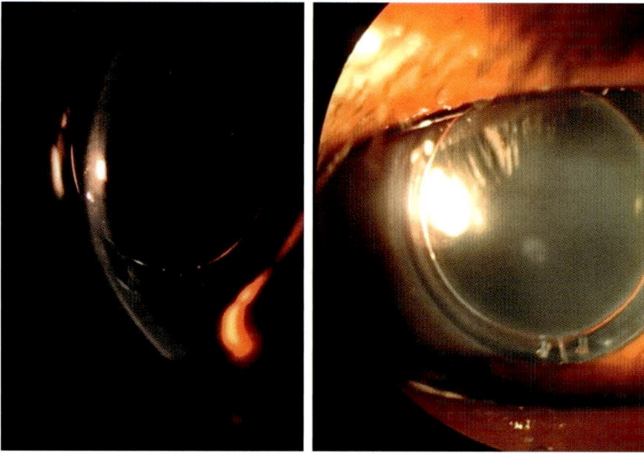

Fig. 2. ICRS placed in the eye of a keratoconic patient using the FS laser technology. The entry cut is obvious and the rings are placed in 70–80% corneal depth.

Commercially Available Intracorneal Ring Segments

At present, three types of ICRSs are available: Intacs (Addition Technologies Inc., Fremont, Calif., USA), Keraring (Mediphacos, Belo Horizonte, Brazil) and Ferrara rings (Ferrara Ophthalmics, Belo Horizonte, Brazil). Ferrara rings have a smaller optical zone and more of a flattening effect than Intacs. New Intacs SK segments have smaller optical zone and thus are more effective in treating severe keratoconus.

Surgical Technique of ICRS Implantation

The mechanical insertion is performed under topical anesthesia. After locating the center of the cornea, a marker is used to mark the sites and the incision points on the steep axis of the cornea. Ultrasound pachymetry is performed to measure the corneal thickness, and a diamond knife is set to a depth between 70 and 80%. A radial incision of 1.2–1.8 mm in width is created in the marked position. Pocketing hooks create corneal pockets on each side at the bottom of the incision. A suction ring is placed around the limbus, and the vacuum system is started. Two semicircular dissectors are placed (one clockwise and the other counterclockwise) into the pocket and are advanced by rotational movement, creating two semicircular tunnels with specific diameters. Ring segments are then placed into the

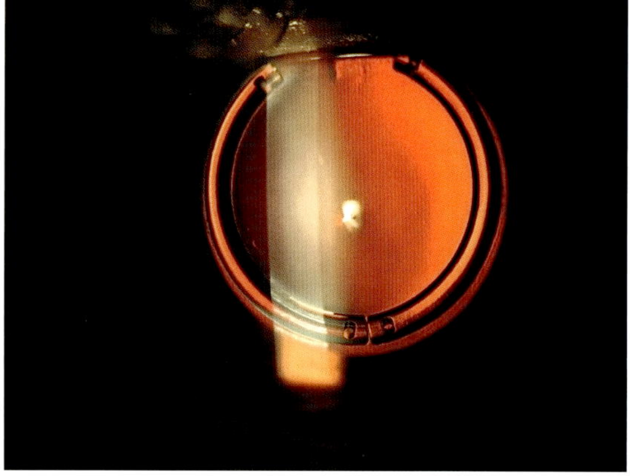

Fig. 3. Slit lamp retroillumination photo of the ICRS in a patient's eye.

tunnels at least 1 mm away from the incision (fig. 2, 3).

The surgical procedure with the FS laser, as in the mechanical procedure, is typically performed under topical anesthesia. After marking a reference point (pupil center or first Purkinje reflex) on the cornea and measuring the corneal thickness by ultrasonic pachymetry at the area of implantation (5- or 6-mm diameter), the disposable suction ring of the FS laser system is centered. The disposable glass lens is applanated to the cornea to fixate the eye and help maintain the precise distance from the laser head to the focal point.

First, an entry cut with the FS laser is created with the aim of allowing access ring placement in the tunnel. The tunnel is then created at approximately 70–80% of the corneal thickness. Afterwards, ring segments are inserted into the created tunnels.

Compared to the manual technique, the FS laser makes tunnel creation faster, easier and more reproducible and it offers accurate tunnel dimensions (width, diameter and depth) [27]. With mechanical dissectors, segment depth may be shallower at positions further from the incision, but it is consistent throughout with the FS laser. Theoretically, as compared with mechanical tunnel creation, which is based on the surgeon's skills, the FS laser-assisted procedure would generate a more accurate stromal dissection leading to better visual and refractive results.

However, similar visual and refractive outcomes with both procedures were reported in a short-term follow-up in keratoconus and post-LASIK ectasia eyes [28, 29].

Kubaloglu et al. [30] compared the clinical outcomes of keratoconic patients treated with Keraring with those treated with Intacs. Both implants were safe and effective. No difference was recorded in visual or refractive outcomes when comparing mechanical and FS laser-created channels. However, they reported that the use of the FS laser made the procedure faster, easier and more comfortable. Of course, further experience and the development of more accurate nomograms should improve clinical outcomes.

Complications of Intracorneal Ring Segment Implantation

Complications associated with the mechanical technique consist of epithelial defects, anterior or posterior perforation with the mechanical spreader, shallow or uneven placement of the ICRSs, decentration, extension of the incision towards the central cornea or limbus and corneal stromal edema around the incision and channel due to surgical manipulation [31, 32]. Most cases of extrusion have been observed in eyes implanted using mechanical dissection, although ring extrusion in advanced keratoconus and segment migration to the incision site have been reported in 3 and 1 case, respectively, using the FS laser-assisted procedure for channel creation [28].

Coskunseven et al. [33] reported the complications after the implantation of intrastromal ring segments in keratoconic patients using the IntraLase FS laser and stated that incomplete channel creation (intraoperatively) and segment migration (postoperatively) were the most common complications. The study demonstrated galvanometer lag error (0.6%), endothelial perforation (0.6%) and vacuum loss (0.1%) as additional intraoperative adverse events and superficial movement of the segments (0.1%), corneal melting (0.2%) and infection (0.1%) as postoperative complications.

Disclosure Statement

Ioannis G. Pallikaris holds the Medical Advisory Board Chair of Presbia (Presbia Flexivue Microlens™).

References

1 Kymionis GD, Bouzoukis DI, Pallikaris IG: Corneal inlays: a surgical correction of presbyopia. J Cat Refr Surg Tod Eur 2007;3:48–50.
2 Barraquer J: Queratoplatica refractiva. Estudios e informaciones. Oftalnologicas 1949;2:10.
3 Choyce P: The present status of intracorneal implants. J Cataract Ophthalmol 1968;3:295.
4 Dohlman C, Refojo M, Rose J: Synthetic polymers in corneal surgery: glyceryl methacrylate. Arch Ophthalmol 1967; 177:52–58.
5 Klyce S, Dingeldein S, Bonanno J, et al: Hydrogel implants: evaluation of first human trial. Invest Ophthalmol Vis Sci Suppl 1988;29:393.

6 Seyeddain O, Riha W, Hohensinn M, et al: Refractive surgical correction of presbyopia with the acufocus small aperture corneal inlay: two-year follow-up. J Refract Surg 2010;26:1–9.

7 Yilmaz O, Bayraktar S, Agca A, et al: Intracorneal inlay for the surgical correction of presbyopia. J Cataract Refract Surg 2008;34:1921–1927.

8 Sharma G, Porter T, Holliday K, et al: Sustainability and biocompatibility of the Presby-Lens corneal inlay for the correction of presbyopia. ARVO 2010; 51:813.

9 Slade ST: Early results using the presbylens corneal inlay to improve near and intermediate vision in emmetropic presbyopes; presented at the ESCRS Annu Meet, Paris, September 2010.

10 Bouzoukis DI, Kymionis GD, Panagopoulou SI, Diakonis VF, Pallikaris AI, Limnopoulou AN, Portaliou DM, Pallikaris IG: Visual outcomes and safety of a small diameter intrastromal refractive inlay for the corneal compensation of presbyopia. J Refract Surg 2012;28:168–173.

11 Limnopoulou AN, Bouzoukis DI, Kymionis GD, Panagopoulou SI, Plainis S, Pallikaris AI, Feingold V, Pallikaris IG: Visual outcomes and safety of a refractive corneal inlay for presbyopia using femtosecond laser. J Refract Surg 2013; 29:12–19.

12 Yilmaz OF, Bayraktar S, Agca A, Yilmaz B, McDonald MB, van de Pol C: Intracorneal inlay for the surgical correction of presbyopia. J Cataract Refract Surg 2008;34:1921–1927.

13 Mulet ME, Alio JL, Knorz MC: Hydrogel intracorneal inlays for the correction of hyperopia: outcomes and complications after 5 years of follow-up. Ophthalmology 2009;116:1455–1466.

14 Verity SM, McCulley JP, Bowman RW, Cavanagh HD, Petroll WM: Outcomes of PermaVision intracorneal implants for the correction of hyperopia. Am J Ophthalmol 2009;147:973–977.

15 Bouzoukis D, Kymionis G, Limnopoulou A, Kounis G, Pallikaris I: Femtosecond laser-assisted corneal pocket creation using a mask for inlay implantation. J Refract Surg 2011;27:818–820.

16 Barraquer JI: Modification of refraction by means of intracorneal inclusions. Int Ophthalmol Clin 1966;6:53–78.

17 Werblin TP, Patel AS, Barraquer JI: Initial human experience with Permalens myopic hydrogel intracorneal lens implants. Refract Corneal Surg 1992;8: 23–26.

18 Alió JL, Mulet ME, Zapata LF, et al: Intracorneal inlay complicated by intrastromal epithelial opacification. Arch Ophthalmol 2004;122:1441–1446.

19 Güell JL, Velasco F, Guerrero E, Gris O, Pujol J: Confocal microscopy of corneas with an intracorneal lens for hyperopia. J Refract Surg 2004;20:778–782.

20 Schanzlin DJ, Asbell PA, Burris TE, Durrie DS: The intrastromal corneal ring segments; phase II results for the correction of myopia. Ophthalmology 1997; 104:1067–1078.

21 Pinero DP, Alio JL, Uceda-Montanes A, et al: Intracorneal ring segment implantation in corneas with postlaser in situ keratomileusis keratectasia. Ophthalmology 2009;116:1665–1674.

22 Pinero DP, Alio JL, Morbelli H, et al: Refractive and corneal aberrometric changes after intracorneal ring implantation in corneas with pellucid marginal degeneration. Ophthalmology 2009;116: 1656–1664.

23 Alio JL, Shabayek MH, Belda JI, et al: Analysis of results related to good and bad outcomes of Intacs implantation for keratoconus correction. J Cataract Refract Surg 2006;32:756–761.

24 Alio JL, Artola A, Ruiz-Moreno JM, et al: Changes in keratoconic corneas after intracorneal ring segment explantation and reimplantation. Ophthalmology 2004;111:747–751.

25 Patel S, Marshall J, Fitzke FWI: Model for deriving the optical performance of the myopic eye corrected with an intracorneal ring. J Refract Surg 1995;11:248–252.

26 Schwartz AR, Tinio BO, Esmail F, Babayan A, Naikoo HN, Asbell PA: Ten-year follow-up of 360 degrees intrastromal corneal rings for myopia. J Refract Surg 2006;22:878–883.

27 Lai MM, Tang M, Andrade EMM, et al: Optical coherence tomography to assess intrastromal ring segment depth in keratoconic eyes. J Cataract Refract Surg 2006;32:1860–1865.

28 Pinero D, Alio L: Intracorneal ring segments in ectatic corneal disease – a review. Clin Experiment Ophthalmol 2010;38:154–167.

29 Rabinowitz YS, Li X, Ignacio TS, Maguen E: Intacs inserts using the femtosecond laser compared to the mechanical spreader in the treatment of keratoconus. J Refract Surg 2006;22:764–771.

30 Kubaloglu A, Cinar Y, Sari ES, et al: Comparison of 2 intrastromal corneal ring segment models in the management of keratoconus. J Cataract Refract Surg 2010;36:978–985.

31 Kanellopoulos AJ, Pe LH, Perry HD, Donnenfeld ED: Modified intracorneal ring segment implantations (Intacs) for the management of moderate to advanced keratoconus; efficiency and complications. Cornea 2006;25:29–33.

32 Boxer Wachler BS, Christie JP, Chandra NS, et al: Intacs for keratoconus. Ophthalmology 2003;110:1031–1040.

33 Coscunseven E, Kymionis GD, Tsiklis NS, et al: Complications of intrastromal corneal ring segment implantation using a femtosecond laser for channel creation: a survey of 850 eyes with keratoconus. Acta Ophthalmol 2011;89:54–57.

Prof. Ioannis G. Pallikaris
Department of Ophthalmology
Medical School, University of Crete
71003 Heraklion, Crete (Greece)
E-Mail pallikar@med.uoc.gr

Subject Index